YOUR KNOWLEDGE HA

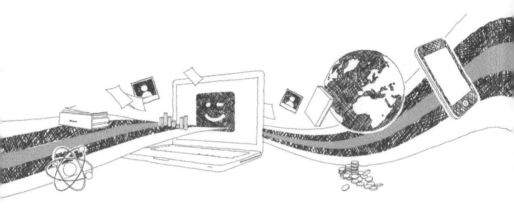

- We will publish your bachelor's and master's thesis, essays and papers

- Your own eBook and book - sold worldwide in all relevant shops

- Earn money with each sale

Upload your text at www.GRIN.com and publish for free

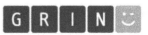

Correlation between Teeth Wear and Oral Health Related Quality of Life among Adult Patients

Rangoli Srivastava

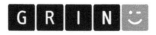

Bibliographic information published by the German National Library:

The German National Library lists this publication in the National Bibliography; detailed bibliographic data are available on the Internet at http://dnb.dnb.de.

ISBN: 9783346910929
This book is also available as an ebook.

© GRIN Publishing GmbH
Trappentreustraße 1
80339 München

Print and binding: Books on Demand GmbH, Norderstedt, Germany
Printed on acid-free paper from responsible sources.

The present work has been carefully prepared. Nevertheless, authors and publishers do not incur liability for the correctness of information, notes, links and advice as well as any printing errors.

GRIN web shop: https://www.grin.com/document/1373671

ACKOWLEDGENT

Though only my name appears on the cover of this dissertation, it wouldn't have been possible without the help and support of a great deal of people.

I extend my heart-felt gratitude to **Dr. Manish Goyal**, Principal and head of the Department of Orthodontics and Dentofacial Orthopaedics for giving me full independence in utilizing all facilities needed to carry out my work.

I owe my sincerest gratitude to my guide, **Dr. Pradeep Tangade** , Professor and head, Department of Public Health Dentistry who has been an excellent teacher. Without his constant concern, support, words of encouragement and constant evaluation this dissertation would have remained just an idea. I also express my gratitude to my faculty *Dr. Thanveer K, Dr. Vikas Singh, Dr. Ankita Jain* for sharing their knowledge & invaluable suggestions.

I am indebted to my parents *Mr. Upendra Kr. Srivastava* and *Mrs. Juhi Srivastava* and my brother *CA Aviral Srivastava* for being my strength and for supporting me in pursuing my dreams. I would not have been where I am today without their guidance, love and support. Their patience and sacrifice will remain my inspiration throughout my life. I also owe my deepest gratitude to my dearest husband *Mr. Shobhit Srivastava* for his eternal support and understanding of my goals and aspirations. His infallible love and support has always been my strength.

I'll also be forever grateful to my grandparents *Dr. Aditya Kumar* and *Mrs. Santosh Srivastava* for their blessings and unconditional love. It is like a drop in the ocean of words that can never reach its mark to acknowledge infinite love, blessings, sacrifices and constant encouragement of my beloved friend *Dr. Vaishali Chaudhary* who have been the sole source of inspiration for me to proceed ahead in my life.

I also extend my gratitude to my in laws, *Mr. Rohit Srivastava, Mrs. Sharmila Srivastava*, and *Sanchit Srivastava* for their constant support and motivation throughout. I also extend my thanks to *Dr. Surbhi Priyadarshi, Dr. Malti, Dr. Priyanshi, Dr. Priya, Dr. Rupali, Dr. Mukul, Dr. Harshita,* for their support.

Above all, I thank, **God Almighty**, who enabled me with philosophy, perception and motivation .

i

LIST OF ABBREVIATIONS

SNO.	ABBREVIATION	FULL FORM
1.	TW	TEETH WEAR
2.	OHRQoL	ORAL HEALTH RELATED QUALITY OF LIFE
3.	QoL	QUALITY OF LIFE
4.	NCCL	NON CARIOUS CERVICAL LESIONS
5.	TSL	TOOTH SURFACE LOSS
6.	OHIP	ORAL HEALTH IMPACT PROFILE
7.	OHIP-14	ORAL HEALTH IMPACT PROFILE(14 QUESTIONNAIRE VERSION)
8.	BEWE	BASIC EROSIVE WEAR EXAMINATION
9.	ETW	EROSIVE TEETH WEAR
10.	CP	CEREBRAL PALSY
11.	P-CPQ	PARENTAL CAREGIVERS PERCEPTION QUESTIONNAIRES
12.	GOHAI	GERIATRIC ORAL HEALTH ASSESSMENT INDEX
13.	OES	OROFACIAL ESTHETIC SCALE
14.	BEWI	BASIC EROSIVE WEAR INDEX
15.	DH	DENTINAL HYPERSENSITIVITY
16.	OIDP	ORAL IMPACT ON DAILY PERFORMANCE
17.	GERD	GASTRO-ORESOPHAGEAL REFLUX DISEASE
18.	OPD	OUT PATIENT DEPARTMENT
19.	PHD	PUBLIC HEALTH DENTISTRY
20.	TMDC & RC	TEERTHANKER MAHAVEER DENTAL COLLEGE AND RESEARCH CENTRE

LIST OF FIGURES

LIST OF TABLES

LIST OF GRAPHS

ABSTRACT

ABSTRACT

INTRODUCTION: Teeth wear can be described as a multi factorial lesion that can affect the quality of life of an individual to a varied extent. Various dietary habits along with various lifestyle habits are associated with this so we need to assess its varied etiology and the effects. Thus this research was conducted in the dental college amongst the age group of 35-44 years participants who were visiting OPD of TMDC & RC, Moradabad.

OBJECTIVES: To assess the prevalence of TW, to assess its impact on OHRQoL and to recommend preventive measures.

MATERIALS AND METHODS: A cross sectional study was conducted in the college of TMDC & RC, Moradabad. Nearly 630 participants were examined clinically for TW. Only those participants were selected who had age between 35-44 years. Informed consent was also obtained from them. Their socio demographic details were noted and along with this their TW was assessed with the help of smith and knight TW index and they also filled a questionnaire of OHIP-14 which was already translated and validated in the Hindi language.

RESULTS: Clinical examination of 630 subjects along with the filling of the OHIP-14 questionnaire by them was done and after examining them we concluded that there is a significantly remarkable association between TW and OHRQoL and TW was also linked to other socio demographic details and various other lifestyle habits and dietary and drinking habits too.

CONCLUSION: With the scope and limitations of this study mentioned, it has thus been concluded that TW has got a direct association and a positive correlation with the OHRQoL. As TW was increasing, so were the OHIP values, which indicated a lesser OHRQoL. Thus this research focuses on the importance of maintaining healthy dietary habits and to treat the TW at an earlier stage.

x

KEY WORDS: Teeth wear, abrasion, attrition, erosion, abfraction.

CONTENTS

INTRODUCTION

Wear is the gradual removal from a matter's surface which is in contact as a result of reference movement at the interface. Wear analysis is a typical procedure for determining the life span of any particle and wear has long been a curious topic in nanostructure materials and materials science. With multiple demographic research showing that dental wearing, particularly erosion, is rising in the normal community, wear emerged as a subject of debate and curiosity amongst dentists.[1]

Teeth wear can be defined as multifaceted, multivariate phenomena which happen as a result of the interaction of various physiological, biomechanical, biochemical, and rheological aspects. The degree of wear of teeth is influenced by things including muscle activity, lubrication, dietary habits, and the kind of restoration done.[2]

Since the dentist particularly has greatest influence over the type of usage of materials, a significant amount of study has focused on enhancing the wear characteristics of materials used in dentistry and thus avoid unnecessary wear on tooth structure.[3]

Wear of teeth can be broadly divided into four categories –

1. Attrition - the deterioration of tooth brought on by contact of one tooth with another tooth during regular or dysfunctional function of masticator muscle.

    Bruxism, which is marked by gripping, crushing, stiffening, or pushing of the lower jaw over a prolonged period of time, is the main key contributor to this phenomenon. This is already acknowledged that this phenomenon can happen while you are sleeping or not sleeping. While sleeping we can call it as sleep bruxism while when one is awake it is referred as awake bruxism. Although the cause of this is uncertain, it is most likely complex involving many factors. All those factors can be as follows – if a person belongs to a younger age group then there are more chances of having bruxism, also females are noted to have had more bruxism as compared to males, those who have a regular and frequent intake of tobacco products, alcohol and caffeine products intake then there are higher chances of having bruxism, most common reason being stressful situations and anxious individuals have a tendency to have bruxism. Some medications also might lead to bruxism. Dentinal layer may become visible as soon as the outermost layer of enamel had been damaged. As a consequence, the area seems to be more prone to more wear. There is frequently a slightly rounded area because to the varying rates of the outermost and second outermost layer deterioration.(Figure-1)

2. Abrasion - pathologic dental wear caused by mechanisms which involve mechanics and friction of tooth with other materials. E.g. this happens while a person brushes his/her teeth. Thus we can say that an external element's contact pressures on a teeth cause this lesion. This could be a behavior, like the tendency to do brushing excessively vigorously or to bite on tough things like stationary and accessories.(Figure-2)

3. Erosion - the external or internal degradation of dental structure resulting from acid breakdown. E.g. damage caused to teeth by regurgitation of gastric acids or by acidic content present in diet. The main factor contributing to wear of teeth as compared to all other types of wear is erosion. It occurs as a consequence of acidic and chemical contents which doesn't have bacterial origin which demineralizes the outermost layer of enamel and further on the second layer's structural organization of crystals present in its framework. There can be many causes of erosion which may be external or internal. Some internal causes include some diseases such as GERD, bulimia nervosa and anorexia nervosa. Those who have an intense habit of having alcohol also suffer from high rate of

erosion. At times dehydration can also be a reason for having erosion. Some external causes of having erosion include high intake of drinks which are carbonated, some fruit based juices and some smoothies, some occupational hazards specifically lead to erosion also people who are associated with sports such as swimming.

Presence of acidic environment could be from an internal source or an external source or may be both can be the reason for etiology of ETW. Wearing on the palatal sides of the upper jaw is a frequent side effect of endogenous acidic dissolution. In such situations, the lower jaw anterior aren't typically affected. Incisal margins of upper jaw anterior may become thinner and more translucent as a consequence of external eroding. Additionally, the surface towards the cheeks and lips along with the surface towards the root of the teeth could also be influenced. As the condition progresses, the outermost surfaces may first show as scooped outward areas all around cuspal tips before taking an increasingly hollow type morphology. Alternately, dryness in mouth due to fewer amounts of water may be the cause of ETW .If a person takes medicines then that also can be a cause of dehydration in a person's mouth.(Figure-3)

4. Abfraction - pathological dental material loss brought about by forces of biomechanical origin. According to some theories, this loss was brought on by the tooth flexing under stress, which fatigued the outermost and second outermost layer away from the area of pressure. Latin origin that meant "to break apart" served as the source of the word "abfraction".[4] (Figure-4)

Erosion (biochemical deterioration caused by internal or external acidity),attrition(loss of tooth layer brought about by adjacent teeth interaction) and abrasion(bodily harm brought on by substances not involving teeth) are three common multivariate causes of dental layer deterioration/wear.[5] Straight, spherical, or highly curved polished areas on the uppermost surfaces of the teeth are known as teeth worn facets, and they could be the consequence of too much grinding of one tooth towards the other tooth.[6] The tooth most usually influenced are lower quadrant posteriors specifically molars and upper quadrant anterior specifically incisors. Both upper and lower arches exhibit both sided and uniform dental wear.[7, 8]

Indices are the most accurate approach to monitor deviation amongst teeth in massive populations. Regardless of the etiology, Smith and Knight developed the broader idea of evaluating worn that has occurred on a tooth per surface. If prevalent at levels over what is deemed normal, tooth wear, a biological phenomenon in and of itself, could have a crippling impact on OHRQoL. The extent up till which any individual appreciates the significant likelihood of having the benefit of life is what is meant by "QoL".

The term "OHRQOL" refers to one's perspective as to how one's dental health affects every aspect of one's life and general health.

The most commonly utilized tool for assessing dental health as well as its effects on people's quality of their living the life is OHIP. Slade created a 14 item questionnaire variant of OHIP-49 because initial OHIP had 49 questions and was built on a conceptual perspective created by WHO which was modified for dental health by Locker. A 14 item checklist with self-reported functional impairment, pain, & impairment due to dental conditions is used to quantify these factors.

Therefore the aim of this dissertation is to find out what is the exact relation between TW and OHRQoL amongst a selected group of participants.

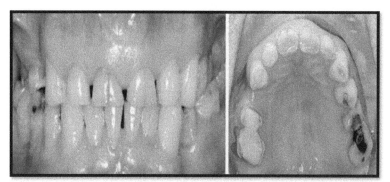

Figure 1 – Attrition(incisal, occlusal surface), Enamel loss

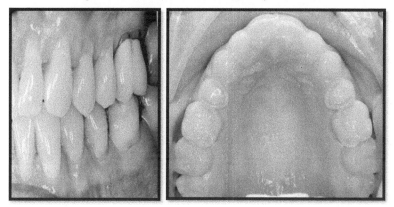

Figure 2 –Abrasion (buccal surface)   Figure 3 – Erosion (palatal surface)

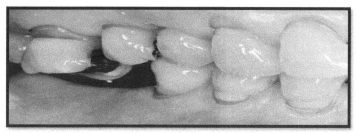

Figure 4 – Abfraction (V-shape appearance)

REVIEW OF

LITERATURE

1. Al-Omiri MK et al (2006)[9] did a research to assess the impact of TW on QoL. For the investigation, seventy six participants with wear of teeth and seventy six placebo had been enrolled. Questionnaire which was used was entitled – Dental Impact on daily living to evaluate the impact of tooth wear on everyday activities and their wellbeing. In a cohort of patients, the extent of tooth wear was evaluated using an ordinal scale. The findings demonstrated that tooth wear had a discernible effect on individuals' happiness with their look, pain thresholds, dental health, overall efficiency, and ability for biting and swallowing. Through the study it was concluded that no matter how severe dental status is, tooth wear has a considerable impact on a participant's contentment with their dental status.

2. Smith WA et al (2007)[10] conducted a study in hospital of Trinidadian University to assess the frequency and intensity of NCCLs in a collective gathering of patients. NCCLs are frequently observed in dental practice, with flexure, erosion, abrasion cited as the causes. This paper aims to determine the prevalence and severity of NCCLs in a sample of patients attending a university clinic in Trinidad and to investigate the relationship with medical and dental histories, oral hygiene practices, dietary habits and occlusion. Data were collected via a questionnaire and clinical examination. Other significant factors included patients who reported heartburn, gastric reflux, headaches, bruxism, sensitive teeth and swimming or had a history of broken restorations in the last year. There was also significant correlation of NCCLs in patients who brushed more than once a day or used a medium or hard toothbrush. Patients with vegetarian diets and those who reported consuming citrus fruits, soft drinks, alcohol, yoghurt and vitamin C drinks were

associated with the presence of lesions. Significant associations were also found in patients with group function, faceting, clicking joints or those who wore occlusal splints.

3. Ahmed H et al (2009)[11] aim to identify contributing factors to NCCLs and the teeth where these lesions occur far more frequently. Study began in 2005 in the month of December and was concluded in 2006 in the month of January in the hospital of the district of Karachi. By using a questionnaire which was pre coded 95 participants with the number of teeth as 671 in total had their dental health examined. Permanent dentition participants who had NCCLs were included. Most of them used a moderate sized brush and a brushed their teeth in horizontal motion. They preferred to brush their teeth two times daily. Majority of them didn't have a habit of Bruxism. Premolars were the teeth most commonly involved with NCCLs. It was most common in middle age people.

4. Wang P et al (2010)[12] gathered a representative sample of 12-13 years school children so as to know what is the relation erosive wear of a tooth with factors that are related to a child's habits related to diet and the beverages intake. Dental erosion is now receiving greater focus as a result of the considerable changes in Chinese culture over through the years. Central incisor's incisal edge was the most prominently involved surface. Females who consumed carbonated drinks suffered from erosion due to this causative factor. This seemed to be a significant problem in that region according to the results of the study.

5. Barlett et al (2011)[13] proposed a design of study to estimate link between intake of food and drinks having acidic content and ETW. Nearly 1010 people having mean age of 21.9 years were evaluated. Amongst them majority were females. Participants were asked to fill a questionnaire which was already validated. It had 50 questions enquiring about their habits related to diet. As per results there was a significant link between habits related to

food intake and drinking water. Also those who possibly had heartburn demonstrated exposure of dentine from palatal side.

6. Al Zarea BK (2012)[14] did an investigation in Saudi Arabia amongst adult population to assess the extent of loss of tooth surface and to assess what are the etiological and associated possible risk factors which increase the chances of causing teeth wear. In this study they took 400 individuals and they were asked to fill a questionnaire and then clinical examination was done to assess the for the extent of TW. Results showed that nearly 3/4th of population had attrition, nearly 90% depicted erosion, nearly 15% depicted abrasion and almost every participant amongst them showed various types of TSL. There was more TW in males. TW had multifactorial causes and amongst them diet was the most evident etiological cause.

7. Papagianni CE et al (2013)[15] evaluated the effect of TW on OHRQoL. There were nearly 198 people included in the study. They were involved with four different types of groups i.e. those having teeth wear, those having painful TMD, patients with complete denture and rest as controls. To assess OHRQoL, OHIP Dutch version was used. Results showed a significant correlation between TW and OHRQoL.

8. Barlett DW et al (2013)[16] proposed a research so that an overall evaluation can be done regarding prevalence of TW on each of tooth surfaces and also to assess possible etiological factors in adults of Europe. Age group that was selected was 18-35 years. Study was done in 3187 participants and evaluation was done for risk factors with a questionnaire which was already validated. Maximum BEWE value for every scoreable surface was used to describe each person. Amongst various countries major differences were seen. Maximum score of TW was seen in UK. Trouble creating factors for TW

included heartburn, continuous episodes of vomiting. There was a positive correlation between uptake of juices, fruits and TW. Nearly 29% showed effects of TW thus representing it as a common finding in adults of Europe.

9. Kumar S et al (2013)[17] did a research in south India amongst children of schools. Age group that was selected was 11-14. Number of participants was 605 and amongst them 302 public school children and 303 private school children were taken. Framing of a questionnaire was done to note details regarding social class, practice regarding oral hygiene, various habits related to diet and possible etiological factors which cause erosion of teeth. In majority of cases (95%) only enamel loss was seen. Though the general prevalence of erosion of teeth was very low (nearly 8.9%). As a result it was seen that the children of private school were comparatively more affected by erosion of teeth.

10. Fotedar S et al (2014)[18] explained OHRQoL amongst adults who visited OPD of PHD department in a dental hospital in Shimla and to find out association between status of dental health and OHRQoL. This study was done for duration of 3 months. This study was conducted amongst 351 participants who reported in college. After this inference was concluded all dental and periodontal findings showed an association with OHRQoL. Thus we can say that OHIP values showed association with dental status.

11. Abanto J (2014)[19] assessed the risk factors associated with ETW specifically amongst children those who are suffering from the disease of cerebral palsy along with impact of TW on OHRQoL were also assessed. According to results, ETW was present in nearly half of children (48.3%). Also it was concluded that one of factors for ETW causation was that they consumed more than 2 days of intake of soft drink in a week, juices which

came in powdered form, therefore as per this study ETW resulted in a negative effect on OHRQoL.

12. Liu B et al (2014)[20] did an analysis amongst adults in north west area of China to assess the occurrence of TW and the associated factors which cause TW. This study was questionnaire based. It included 704 adults. Study was done on participants who visited the hospital for routine examination. Also it was concluded through the study that TW is caused due to dietary factors. Therefore this study concluded that there is a relation between TW and diet pattern.

13. Visscher CM et al (2014)[21] assessed relation between dental status and OHRQoL in a population. This study was done in a population of 1622 participants. Clinical examination was done and questionnaire was filled by them. For recording OHRQoL they used Dutch version of OHIP questionnaire. As per results there was a significant level of difference between various dental status groups. Also it was concluded that impeded dental status was directly related to worsening OHRQoL.

14. Pradeep Y, Pushpanjali K (2014)[22] assessed the influence of dental health on QoL amongst patients who are visiting dental hospitals and private dental clinic. Questionnaire that was used was OHRQoL. Nearly 1200 participants whose age group was more than 16 years were selected with the help of sampling. As per results nearly 78% of participants seemed to have their QoL. Those who belonged to lower social class amongst them women believed that oral health of theirs was comparatively negative as compared to those of higher class.

15. Kumar S et al (2015)[23] assessed the prevalence and associated factors of NCCLs amongst children who belong to special needs. Numbers of participants were 395. They belonged

to age group of 12-15 years. Results showed that because of usage of tooth powder or different ways of cleaning their teeth, comparatively tough bristles, horizontal brushing pattern, diet purely vegetarian and increased uptake of citric items lead to NCCLs. Nearly 22.7% of population was affected by NCCLs.

16. Hegde MN, Nireeksha (2015)[24] determined prevalence of TW because of diet related factors amongst people of South Canada. This study was conducted in a duration of 1 month in the city of Mangalore. Nearly 58.7% of population had TW with most of them having abrasion, attrition, abfraction followed by erosion. Males had considerably more TW as compared to females. Non vegetarians had considerably more TW as compared to vegetarians. Most TW was seen in age group of 56-65 years. Specifically in age group of 26-35 years erosion was seen(alcohol being the major reason for that). Hence through this study it was concluded that dietary factors plays a major role in causation of TW.

17. Deshpande S (2015)[25] evaluated severity, prevalence and knowledge amongst adult patients who visited dental college's hospital in Nagpur. A questionnaire was used which was already validated to assess occurrence, severity of TW. Along with TW, dentinal hypersensitivity and other oral habits were also assessed. Nearly 570 participants had their clinical examination done in which both males and females were there. Age group of 25-55 years was taken. Those who had TW 1 or 2 didn't have proper knowledge and were not aware of TW. Those who had grade 3 TW were having more awareness and those who had TW 4 their awareness was double as compared to grade 3.

18. Andrade FJ et al (2015)[26] determined relation amongst nutritional intake, wear of teeth and the quality of life of those children of school in brazil. Nutritional intake of a child was calculated with anthropometry with the help of BMI evaluation and TW was

assessed with the help of indices of TW. After recording BMI it was seen that nearly $1/3^{rd}$ of boys and girls were underweight. It was seen that those who were overweight had more TW in deciduous teeth while there was more TW in permanent teeth of obese children. Also there was correlation between age and TW.

19. Sanadhaya S et al (2015)[27] evaluated psychometric characteristics regarding OHIP-14 amongst population of Udaipur's rural and urban population and to evaluate dental status and effect on OHRQoL. OHIP-14 showed significant association with demographic details and also with number of missing and decayed teeth. Odds ratio was higher in males and urban population. Dental caries also had valuable effect on OHRQoL.

20. Li MHM, Bernabe E (2016)[28] came up with a correlation between TW and OHRQoL amongst population of adults in UK. Nearly 5654 individuals were evaluated for wear of teeth. Further their TW severity was divided into mild, moderate, severe. OHIP was recorded with the help of shorter version of OHIP-14. It was seen that those individuals who had severe TW had a high OHIP-14 score. If we assess for domain then psychological discomfort had most high score. Therefore there was a direct association of OHIP-14 score being higher along with severe TW. Hence it was concluded that TW was associated in a negative way with psychological effect in lives of people.

21. Antunes LAA et al (2016)[29] assessed risk factors which are related to bruxism and further finding affect of bruxism on OHRQoL in children aged 3-6 years. Those children were taken from preschools which were public from Brazil. There were case group and control group there were 21 students in case and 40 students in control group. There seemed no statistical significant association between bruxism's presence or absence or rest variables. Therefore we can conclude that bruxism of these children seemingly associated with

issues of respiratory system, wear of teeth, carious teeth and malocclusion of teeth. Irrespective of the fact that bruxism demands proper attention in dental, bruxism seemingly didn't impacted OHRQoL significantly.

22. Masood M et al (2016)[30] examined factors that determine OHRQoL amongst people who were old in age in the country of UK. Population that was chosen were those who belonged to an age group of more than 65 years. As per older studies there was a medium relation between QoL and dental diseases in a survey conducted on a larger scale. Because there were caries that led to poor OHRQoL in aged people, but it didn't indicated their periodontal health. Main conclusion came out to be that along with aiming at prevention of any disease there is a continuous need for regular screening along with treatment in assessed population.

23. Vidyadhar MSB et al (2017)[31] examined link between diet a person takes and if his/her habits related to diet were related to TW or not. This study was done in adults in age group of 18-30 years. For selecting cases, those participants were selected who were having TW. Clinical examination included assessment of TW with simplified TW index given by Bardsley in 2004. As per results it was seen that TW was more in cases. It was seen that cases had more fruits, drinks which were carbonated foods which were carbonated foods which were acidic, products composed of tobacco and also their brushing pattern was incorrect along with these habits they also used toothbrush with hard bristles hence concluding the reason for their TW.

24. Al-Allaq T et al (2018)[32] determined range to which an association might be there between TW and QoL in participants who are local residents of nursing home. Examiner investigated extent of TW in each of them as per adapted TW index of Donachie & Walls

and then further verbally enquired regarding GOHAI. As per results there wasn't any statistical significant demarcation between male and female TW but TW was positively associated to age and negatively associated to QoL.

25. Praveena J et al (2018)[33] found out how many people are affected with TW and how TW has an effect on OHRQoL. Along with TW measurement its impact on OHRQoL was also assessed in those participants who had considerable TW. As per results it was seen that nearly 40% participants had score of 2 in TW and nearly 20% participants had a score of 3 in TW. After measuring all dimensions mean OHIP came out to be 16.91 and nearly 36.7% population had moderately affected effect on OHRQoL. TW severity was 2 and with medium effect on OHRQoL.

26. Hegde M et al (2018)[34] assessed occurrence of TW in south west participants from and to identify various associated factors. This study happened in Mangalore. Nearly 1000 participants were assessed if they had physiological types of TW and along with this a questionnaire which helped them assess various etiological factors linked with TW. 40-60 years aged people had more TW. Males had comparatively more TW. Erosion was seen to be more in those participants who took alcohol and aerated drinks. Attrition was more in those participants who consumed tobacco on a daily basis and also those who had a habit of bruxism. Thus through this study we saw extent of TW and associated etiologies of that TW in that population.

27. Sterenborg B A M M et al (2018)[35] determined range of OHRQoL and how their oral and facial structures appeared in participants who had TW in range of moderate and severe. The advisory group showed that their values didn't change after an year. If we assess restorative group, in them values got better in that year. Thus we can say that only

counseling patients and monitoring them doesn't bring any improvement in QoL. Rather restorative treatment is a better option.

28. Kumar A et al (2019)[36] determined association between erosion 400 occupational workers had because of their profession and OHRQoL. This study was conducted in factory workers of Bangalore. OHIP-14 was used to assess their OHRQoL. Almost half of population showed positive work practice related to behavior. Dental erosion was more in study group. OHIP score was less in study group. As a conclusion we can say that dental erosion was associated with occupation and OHIP-14.

29. Mehta SB et al (2020)[37] evaluated association between TW range. Nearly 319 participants were involved in the study and they were assessed by conducting a BEWE on them. Participants were taken from various other places of UK, Australia, and Malta. For assessing impact on QoL. Mean BEWE score came out to be nearly 6.7. OHIP came out to be nearly 1.84. There seemed to be a significant relationship between BEWE score rise and OHIP score in total. In the end we can conclude that as TW is raising it led to worsening OHRQoL.

30. Patel J, Baker SR (2020)[38] assessed relationship in TW and OHRQoL amongst adult population of UK. Nearly 5187 people were assessed for TW by conducting a survey of dental health of adults. As a result we could see that there was a significant relation between TW and OHRQoL. As TW was increasing impact of TW on daily living measured by OHIP was increasing. Individuals who were young seemed to have more secure impact on OHIP. Concluding thus that we can say that in such a large population there was a significantly less relation between TW & OHRQoL.

31. Al-Khalifa KS (2020)[39] found occurrence of TW in Saudi Arabia amongst adults and also to find out associated etiological factors e.g. socio economic status and demographic details. Nearly 83.5% population was affected by TW and nearly 58.8% had their dentin exposed. As per results sex and level of education showed a significant relation with TW. It was more in population. If we find out causes of TW, it can lead to prevention of severe symptoms and associated rising TW.

32. Soares ARDS et al (2021)[40] evaluated relation between hypersensitivity of dentine and both psychosocial and physical oral health impact. It was conducted in Brazil over the span of an year. Both interview and clinical examination was done by examiners who were calibrated and trained. NCCLs assessment was done by measuring TWI with the help of a probe. Nearly 197 adults were assessed. Out of them more than half of population had impact on oral health. More impact on oral health was seen in those adults who had dental hypersensitivity; more impact on specific pain dimension was seen amongst other dimensions. Dentinal hypersensitivity seemed to have more oral health impact.

33. Kalsi H et al (2021)[41] determined association between QoL both specific and general wellbeing personality in participants having TW. Participants belonging to a age group 18 till 70 years were selected. Those participants were selected who were having TW. Those who were having higher BEWE score were further associated with older age and even worse QoL. After doing analysis of all variables, linear regression we came up with conclusion that QoL insight is a bit complicated and just TW increase is not the only factor which can lead to a decrease on QoL

34. Penoni DC et al (2021)[42] investigated etiological reasons for NCCLs so that proper anticipation of NCCL can be done. This study also aimed to find out occurrence of NCCL. Nearly 501 people were analyzed. Nearly 62.5% population was affected by NCCLS. Amongst an age group of 15-39 years, males were having more NCCL especially those males who had less teeth and diet which had more acidic content. Thus NCCL was associated with demographic details, dental status, brushing patterns.

35. Kanaan M et al (2022)[43] assessed the range till where the altered for indicating related to health effects OHRQoL in adults. Nearly 570 adults were evaluated. Those adults were taken at an age of more than 18 years. Those individuals were selected who had molar contact on both sides. Participants gave answers to the questionnaire in which four different areas were covered. Results also showed that those who belonged to age group of 35-44 years who didn't receive proper dental care, who took carbonated drinks, whose teeth were sensitive and those who thought that morphologically their teeth have altered demonstrated lesser OHRQoL. Though we can say that TW was high in population but its effect on OHRQoL was less.

36. Lim SN et al (2022)[44] did an investigation on ETW occurrence and linked etiological factors amongst younger army professionals in country of Singapore. TW was assessed by BEWE index. Amongst them nearly 21% had TW. Etiological factors were GERD, TMD symptoms, food having acidic content, carbonated drinks, caries, hard toothbrush bristles. Therefore because a high population was at risk so everyone should be educated at a young age.

AIM AND
OBJECTIVES

AIM

To correlate TW & OHRQoL amongst adult patients aged 35-44 years attending TMDC&RC, Moradabad, Uttar Pradesh, India.

OBJECTIVES

1. To assess the prevalence of teeth wear among adult patients aged 35-44 years visiting OPD of college.
2. To assess the oral health related quality of life among adult patients aged 35-44 years visiting OPD of college.
3. To assess the effect of teeth wear on oral health related quality of life among adult patients aged 35-44 years visiting OPD of college.
4. To recommend preventive measures.

MATERIAL AND

METHODS

The purpose of the current research was to evaluate the correlation between TW and OHRQoL among adult patients aged 35-44 years attending OPD of TMDC&RC, Moradabad, Uttar Pradesh, India

1. STUDY AREA

The district of Moradabad is located to the northwest of Lucknow, the state capital of U.P. TMDC&RC is an institutional and research centre located in district of Moradabad, Uttar Pradesh. Moradabad district has a total area of 349.9 square kilometers, as of the 2011 Census with a total population of 889,819. In total male population was about 15, 01,927 and females are 12, 49,094.Literacy rate is 58.67%.

2. SOURCE OF DATA

The present study will be carried amongst the adult patients attending OPD of TMDC&RC. A standardized, closed-ended questionnaire was used to gather information, and then participants in the study underwent an oral clinical evaluation.

3. STUDY POPULATION

Adult patients aged 35-44 years attending OPD of TMDC&RC were included in this cross-sectional study.

4. PILOT STUDY

It was done before beginning main study amongst fifty participants who fulfilled the eligibility criteria.35-44 year aged subjects were selected and examined according to the criteria set for the study and the demographic profile was also recorded.

The information from survey (pilot) was excluded from the final research and proforma of the main study was modified as needed in light of the findings.

5. SAMPLING PROCEDURE

For estimating sample size of this study we took the help of the pilot survey we did and also the preceding researches that were conducted.

Following formula was used for calculating value of sample size.

Size of sample (N) is $\dfrac{Z^2PQ}{L^2}$

Z refers to Normal Distribution's point, taken in accordance with a table in which as per normal curve the interval of confidence selected was 95% and hence the value is 1.96

P refers to Interest's proportion which is 37.97%

Q refers to prevalence (alternate) which is 62.03

L refers to 10% of prevalence which is 3.8

$$N= \dfrac{(1.96)^2\,37.97\times62.0}{(3.8)^2} = 624$$

624 is sample size but taking non-response rate, error, drop-size, attrition into consideration, 650 was taken as final sample size.

6. INCLUSION CRITERIA:

- Adult patients aged 35-44 years attending OPD of TMDC&RC
- Adult patients who are interested by themselves to take part in the research and who gave informed consent.

7. EXCLUSION CRITERIA:

- Adult patients with apparent medical/oral conditions(excluding tooth wear)

- Adult individuals who declined to take part in the research

- Adult patients who are suffering from any systemic disease

- Adult patients who are undergoing orthodontic treatment

8. ETHICAL CLEARANCE

The ethical committee received approval to conduct the research of TMDC&RC Committee and the reference number assigned was TMDCRC/IEC/20-21/PHD2 **(Annexure I)**

9. INFORMED CONSENT

Signed informed consent was obtained from each participant and only those who willingly gave the informed consent were included in the study. **(Annexure II)**

10. SCHEDULING

This cross sectional survey was scheduled for a period of 3 months.

11. TRAINING AND CALIBRATION

By doing the test, the examiners were educated beforehand and calibration was already done on the predetermined individuals two times, with half an hour gap between each in department of Public Health Dentistry.

12. RECORDING CLERK

The examiner was accompanied by one recording clerk who was also a dentist to note down the information collected during examination and was well versed with the indices used and coding systems. The recording clerk was calibrated and standardized with the scoring criteria and coding system of the research based indices. Prior to primary research's beginning, the clerks were made to practice the recording of findings during pilot study and mistakes and omissions were rectified.

13. ARMAMENTARIUM:

The following instruments and supplies will be used:

➤ Mouth Mirror

➤ Explorer

➤ Tweezers

➤ Kidney trays

➤ Disposable mouth masks

➤ Disposable gloves

➤ Sanitizer

➤ Sterile gauze

➤ Cotton holders

➤ Cotton gauges

➤ Head cap

➤ Hand wash

➤ Instrument pouch

➤ Hand Towels

➤ OHIP-14 Questionnaire

➤ Data recording sheets, pen and pencils

14. INFECTION CONTROL

Proper measures and standard protocols were followed in order to control infection during survey procedure. The instruments to be utilized for examination were sterilized prior to the initiation of the survey procedure. Dispensable gloves and mouth mask were used by the investigator during assessment of the oral cavity. Oral examination was done by the researcher using all required instruments. Ample sets of instruments were carried to ensure that every single instrument was used just for once.

A separate container was used to store the used instruments. The area was cleaned using the surface disinfectants where the examination was carried out. The collected waste was later disposed off in the hospitals by using appropriate waste disposal technique. Because of this study conducted right after covid-19 pandemic, all these processes were carried out following covid-19 protocols.

15. COLLECTION OF DATA

Regarding purpose of gathering all the necessary and pertinent details, a previously tested questionnaire along with proforma created in native mode of communication were employed.

The questionnaire was based on collection of details regarding demographic details, details related to the category of socioeconomic status to which they belong, their daily habits and practices related to oral hygiene, how many times they visited a dentist or a dental clinic etc. raising enquiry about one's own told dental health and hygiene state and a set of 14 questions which were related to OHRQoL.

All patients aged 35-44 years attending dental outpatient department who fulfilled the inclusion criteria were included in the study. The questionnaires which were used were translated versions of the questionnaire for the convenience of the patient. All the subjects selected for the study were clinically examined and were asked to fill the questionnaires. For the illiterate or low educated patients questions were read by the investigator in the same manner to avoid any bias and the patient was guided through the options to choose a specific response. Demographic details of the patient included general details, habits related to oral hygiene like how many times they visited a dentist or a dental clinic, oral hygiene and material used frequency of brushing, consumption of fruit /citric drinks, consumption of beverages /carbonated drinks and the type of brushing technique used. **(Annexure-III)**

General information compromised of socioeconomic status. Socio-economic status had been classified according to Modified B.G. Prasad's classification, Updated 2020. As per the classification of this particular unit the population is divided into following classes based upon education, occupation and family income.

The original classification of socio-economic status (1961)[45]

Approximate Equivalent Socioeconomic Category	Percapita Family Income Rs Per Month
Upper class	More than Rs100
Class of upper middle range	Rs 50 to Rs 99
Class of lower middle range	Rs 30 to Rs 49
Class of upper lower range	Rs 15 to Rs 29
Class of lower range	Minimum than Rs 15

To update following classification the following formula was used:

Category of the class to which the population belong= Value of CPI of the year × 4.93 / 100

Where, CPI refers to the consumer price index

4.93= Factor of multiplication, It converts the CPI's actual prices into fictitious figures of comparing the CPI to baseline period belonging to year 1961.

Prasad's socioeconomic categorization has already been amended for the year 2020[45]

Category of social class	Updated for the year 2020(depicted in the range of Rs per month)
Category I social class	Range higher than 7533
Category II social class	Range between Rs 7532 and Rs 3766
Category III social class	Range between Rs 3765 and Rs 2260
Category IV social class	Range between Rs 2259 and Rs 1130
Category V social class	Range lower than 1129

Annual income was then obtained from subjects and divided by 12 (months) and then the value was divided by the number of family members to get the per capita income of the family. This percapita income was subjected to the modified Prasad's classification. Prevalence of teeth wear will be assessed using Smith and Knight TW index. **(ANNEXURE-IV)**

SMITH AND KNIGHT TW INDEX[46]

All the present and seen areas of every tooth existing are assessed for wearing in this index, regardless of how the wearing happened. Four surfaces normally present are the buccal or the labial surface, cervical surface, lingual or the palatal surface and the occlusal or incisal surface. Due to the presence of cervical groove deficiencies in certain individuals, which may not be related to wear present on the cheek side i.e. buccal side overall and could have a distinct causation, thus even the buccal and cervical area/surface's wear are documented independently. For a person having 32 teeth in his/her oral cavity there come out $32 \times 4 = 128$ surfaces recorded in total. Teeth which are absent or are congenitally missing and extensive restoration surfaces are not recorded. The index may be documented either by visual examination or through images. The basic TW scores could be used in a variety of analyses to create profiles of TW pattern for particular participants with recognized shared etiologies, for various different demographic sub-groups, also for separate individuals.

ALLOTTED SCORE*	ASSESSED AREA OF THAT TOOTH	STANDARD CRITERIA FOR DESIGNATING SCORE
0	B , L, O, I C	Zero deterioration of the outermost layer properties Zero change in shape
1	B, L, O, I C	Alterations/deficit in outermost layer properties Very less change in shape
2	B, L, O I	Outermost layer breakdown that exposes second outermost layer on not greater than 30 percent of the total surface outermost layer deficit with exposure of second

		layer of dentine
	C	lesion having a depth of not more than 1 mm
3	B, L, O	enamel thinning that exposes layer of dentine on more than 30% of the area
	I	reduction in the layer of enamel and significant reduction in the layer of dentine
	C	lesions not having a depth greater or in excess of 1-2 mm
4	B, L, O	lesions specifically belonging to outermost layer in its entirety, exposed innermost pulp and subsequent exposed layer of dentin
	I	Exposed layer of secondary dentine or even of the innermost pulp
	C	Defect more than 2mm deep-pulp exposure-secondary dentine exposure. Lesions having a depth greater than 2 mm along with large exposed pulp and secondary layer of dentine

*A lesser value is provided if there is any ambiguity.

B indicates buccal/labial surface

L indicates lingual/palatal surface

O indicates occlusal surface

I indicates incisal surface

C indicates cervical surface

The already translated form of of the OHIP instrument will be used to measure the effect of TW on OHRQoL. (**ANNEXURE-V**)

OHRQoL QUESTIONNAIRE[47]

Different techniques are utilized to assess the influence of alterations in OHRQoL on dentistry related results. The most popular technique for determining OHRQoL parameters is OHIP-14. It illustrates how dental diseases have quite an effect on individual's overall health. The seven theoretically stated components of Locker's conceptual perspective of dental healthcare provide the basis for around 49 items in OHIP-14. In circumstances in which the original version having forty nine questions is unsuitable, 14 question versions were created as a condensed form. Duration of range for which they need to answer the questions could be 12 months. The values of this scale range from 0 till 56 for those 14 questions and as the scale rises it depicts a comparatively low OHRQoL. This scale of OHIP-14 was changed from English to native language version as per proper criteria.

It is a self-reported questionnaire with an emphasis on seven impact factors. The seven domains being as follows-

1. The first domain describes the limitations that a person faces function wise, this particular domain is designated as functional limitation.

2. The second domain describes the pain that a person bears physically; this particular domain is designated as physical pain.

3. The third domain describes the discomfort that a person faces psychologically; this particular domain is designated as psychological discomfort.

4. The fourth domain describes the disability that a person faces physically; this particular domain is designated as physical disability.

5. The fifth domain describes the disability that a person psychologically, this particular domain is designated as psychological disability.

6. The sixth domain describes the disability that a person faces socially; this particular domain is designated as social disability.

7. The seventh domain describes the conditions related to the feeling of handicap in a person.

Amongst options available, there are 5 scores on the scale in which individuals are required to reply/mark the options based on their opinions. They give a score of zero when their opinion is never, a score of one when their opinion goes for hardly ever, a score of two when their opinion is occasionally, a score of three when their opinion is fairly often, a score of four when their opinion is very often.

OHIP-14 HINDI TRANSLATION[48]

With the aid of method of back translation to equalize social aspect, OHIP-14 was modified in both ways (as per language and as per ethnicity). Whatever differences came out in between translated version and original version of OHIP were further checked and evaluated, thus proving the point that both the versions are more or less same. The rechecked version of OHIP-14 Hindi is appropriate to be taken for any pilot study.

16. STATISTICAL ANALYSIS:

Two phases were required to complete the statistical process-

1. Gathering and representation of data

2. Research of statistical data and analysis

The data obtained was compiled systematically from a pre-coded proforma in computer and a master table was prepared. Utilizing SPSS 20th version, the data evaluation was carried out. Continuous measure's outcomes are given in the pattern of Mean±SD (Min-Max) categorical measure's outcomes were given in the pattern of Number (%).The level of significance of 5% was used to determine relevance.

These statistics algorithms were employed:

i) Mean

The average, often known as the mean, is the sum of N.

$$\overline{X} = \frac{\Sigma X}{N}$$

Where:

$\overline{X}$ Refers to the mean of set of details

Σ indicates total

X refers to the values present in distribution; N refers to the distribution score values

ii) Standard Deviation (N)

The Standard deviation is used to measure Variability. The standard deviation is denoted by SD. It can be defined as specifically root square of aggregate of all measured deviations from observations' mean.

$$SD = \sqrt{\frac{\Sigma(X - \bar{X})^2}{N}}$$

Easy formula for calculation of SD

$$SD = \sqrt{\frac{\Sigma X^2 - \frac{(\Sigma X)^2}{N}}{N}}$$

When,

Σ indicates total

X refers to the value obtained

$\bar{X}$ Indicates data's score (mean)

N indicates value frequency

iii) Chi square test

It is an alternate method of measuring the substantial difference between two or more than two proportions

$$\chi^2 = \Sigma \frac{(O-E)^2}{E}$$

When:

O indicates the frequency which is observed

E indicates the frequency which is observed

iv) ANOVA

This assessment is used to assess the null hypothesis that is used to verify the difference in statistical values between one or more independent groups. This compares the means among the groups

The formula for the one-way **ANOVA** F-test statistic is

$$F = \frac{\text{between-group variability}}{\text{within-group variability}}.$$

The variability present between two or more groups" is

$$\sum_{i=1}^{K} n_i(\bar{Y}_{i.} - \bar{Y})^2/(K-1)$$

When

Y_i indicates mean of the sample,

n_i indicates observation number,

$\bar{Y}$ indicates collective data mean,

K indicates group frequency.

The "within-group variability" is

$$\sum_{i=1}^{K}\sum_{j=1}^{n_i}(Y_{ij} - \bar{Y}_{i.})^2/(N-K),$$

Where, Yij is the jth observation in the ith out of K groups and N is the overall sample size.

v) Post Hoc Tukey–

It is a test used to determine whether discrepancies among two different groups' means are meaningfully different. When we want to contrast the means of two groups in pairs and provided sample size is same among both groups. If the sample size is unequal in both groups then other assessments are used.

$$HSD = q \sqrt{\frac{MS_{within}}{n}}$$

q = standardized range statistic

MS_{within}= mean square for within groups from the Anova

n = number of subjects within each group

vi) Level of significance

If the value of level of significance comes out to be less than 0.005 it indicates association which is noteworthy.

If the value of level of significance comes out to be greater than 0.005 it indicates non-significance.

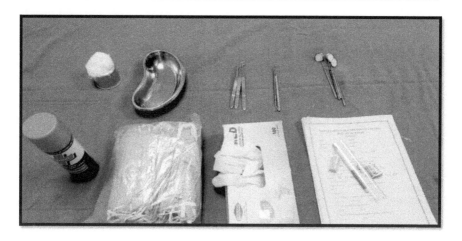

Figure 5 – Armamentarium used

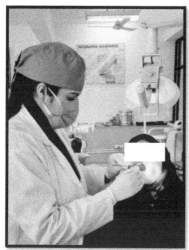 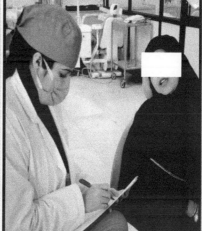

Figure 6 – Clinical examination   Figure 7 – Recording data

RESULTS

For finding out correlation between TW and OHRQoL among 35-44 years patients visiting TMDCRC, Moradabad, Uttar Pradesh, the final sample size came out to consist of 630 subjects.

GENDER DISTRIBUTION OF STUDY SUBJECTS

In study population of 630 participants 343(54.4%) were male in the age group 35-44 years and 287(45.6%) were female in the age group of 35-44 years. (Table-1, Graph-1)

ASSOCIATION OF STUDY SUBJECTS WITH GENDER ON TEETH-WEAR

Amongst a study population having 340 males, majority of males i.e. 228(66.5%) had TW ranging from 2 to 3, then nearly 97(28.27%) males had TW ranging from 1-2 and nearly 18(5.24%) had TW ranging from 3-4.And amongst a study population having 287 females, majority of females i.e. 169(58.88%) had TW ranging from 2 to 3, then nearly 112(39.02%) females had TW ranging from 1-2 and nearly 6(2.09%) had TW ranging from 3-4. A significantly significant relationship was discovered between gender and TW when value of significance came out to be 0.004. (Table-14, Graph-14)

AGE DISTRIBUTION OF STUDY PARTICIPANTS

In study population of 630 participants, 35-44 age group people were selected. Out of them 52(8.3%) participants were of 35 years, 60(9.5%) participants were of 36 years, 69(11.0%) participants were of 37 years, 103(16.3%) participants were of 38 years, 62(9.8%) participants were of 39 years, 86(13.7%) participants were of 40 years, 49(7.8%) participants were of 41 years, 70(11.1%) participants were of 42 years, 39(6.2%) participants were of 43 years, 34(5.4%) participants were of 44 years, 6(1%) participants were of 45 years. Mean age of participants came out to be 39.2±2.623. (Table-2, Graph-2)

ASSOCIATION OF STUDY SUBJECTS WITH AGE ON TEETH-WEAR

Amongst a study population of age group ranging from 35-44 years, In the age group of 35 years,29(55.8%) of participants had TW ranging from 2-3, and 23(44.2%) had TW ranging from 1-2. In the age group of 36 years,32(53.3%) of participants had TW ranging from 2-3, and 28(46.7%) had TW ranging from 1-2.In the age group of 37 years,40(58%) of participants had TW ranging from 2-3, and 23(33.3%) had TW ranging from 1-2 and just 6(8.7%) had TW ranging from 3-4.In the age group of 38 years,56(54.4%) of participants had TW ranging from 2-3, and 35(34%) had TW ranging from 1-2 and just 12(11.7%) had TW ranging from 3-4.In the age group of 39 years,30(48.4%) of participants had TW ranging from 2-3, and 32(51.6%) had TW ranging from 1-2. In the age group of 40 years,71(82.6%) of participants had TW ranging from 2-3, and 15(17.4%) had TW ranging from 1-2.In the age group of 41 years,37(75.5%) of participants had TW ranging from 2-3, and 12(24.5%) had TW ranging from 1-2.In the age group of 42 years,34(48.6%) of participants had TW ranging from 2-3, and 30(42.9%) had TW ranging from 1-2, and just 6(8.6%) had TW ranging from 3-4.In the age group of 43 years,34(87.2%) of participants had TW ranging from 2-3, and 5(12.8%) had TW ranging from 1-2.In the age group of 44 years,28(82.4%) of participants had TW ranging from 2-3, and 6(17.6%) had TW ranging from 1-2.In the age group of 45 years,6(100%) of participants had TW ranging from 2-3. A significantly significant relationship was discovered between groupings of age and TW when value of significance came out to be 0.004. (Table-14, Graph-14)

DISTRIBUTION OF STUDY PARTICIPANTS AS PER SOCIOECONOMIC STATUS

Amongst study population of 630 participants, 42(6.7%) participants belonged from upper class, 88(14%) belonged from upper middle class, 222(35.2%) participants belonged from lower middle class, 205(32.5%) participants belonged from upper lower class, 73(11.6%) participants belonged from lower class. (Table-3, Graph-3)

ASSOCIATION OF STUDY SUBJECTS WITH SOCIO-ECONOMIC STATUS ON TEETH-WEAR

Amongst the study population belonging from upper class, majority of participants (88.1%) had TW ranging from 2-3 and 5(11.9%) participants had TW ranging from 1-2. Amongst the study population belonging from upper middle class, majority of participants (46.6%) had TW ranging from 1-2 and 35(39.8%) participants had TW ranging from 2-3 and just 12(13.6%) participants had TW ranging from 3-4.Amongst the study population belonging from lower middle class, majority of participants (72.1%) had TW ranging from 2-3 and 56(25.2%) participants had TW ranging from 1-2 and just 6(2.7%) participants had TW ranging from 3-4. Amongst the study population belonging from upper lower class, majority of participants (56.1%) had TW ranging from 2-3 and 84(41%) participants had TW ranging from 1-2 and just 6(2.9%) participants had TW ranging from 3-4.Amongst the study population belonging from lower class, majority of participants (68.5%) had TW ranging from 2-3 and 23(31.5%) participants had TW ranging from 1-2. A significantly significant relationship was discovered between socioeconomic status and TW when value of significance came out to be 0.002. (Table 14, Graph-15)

DISTRIBUTION OF STUDY PARTICIPANTS AS PER PLACE OF RESIDENCE

Amongst study population of 630 participants of Moradabad, 159(25.2%) participants belonged from village while 471(74.8%) participants were inhabitants of city. (Table-4, Graph-4)

ASSOCIATION OF STUDY SUBJECTS WITH PLACE OF RESIDENCE ON TEETH-WEAR

Amongst village residents nearly 55(34.6%) participants had TW ranging from 1-2, 92(57.9%) had TW ranging from 2-3, 12(7.5%) participants had TW ranging from 3-4.Amongst city residents nearly 154(32.7%) participants had TW ranging from 1-2, 305(64.8%) had TW ranging from 2-3, 12(2.5%) participants had TW ranging from 3-4. A significantly insignificant relationship was discovered between residence of a person and TW when value of significance came out to be 0.012. (Table 14, Graph-15)

DISTRIBUTION OF STUDY PARTICIPANTS AS PER EDUCATIONAL QUALIFICATION

Amongst study population of 630 participants, 57(9%) participants were 10th pass, 144(24.9%) participants were 12th pass, 384(61%) participants were 12th pass, and 45 (7.1%) participants were post graduates. (Table-5, Graph-5)

ASSOCIATION OF STUDY SUBJECTS WITH EDUCATIONAL QUALIFICATION ON TEETH-WEAR

Amongst 10th pass participants, 17(29.8%) participants had TW ranging from 1-2, 40(70.2%) participants had TW ranging from 2-3.Amongst 12th pass participants, 67(46.5%) participants had TW ranging from 1-2, 71(49.3%) participants had TW ranging from 2-3, 6(4.2%) participants had TW ranging from 3-4.Amongst graduate participants, 125(32.6%) had TW ranging from 1-2, 247(64.3%) participants had TW ranging from 2-3, 12(3.1%) participants had TW ranging from 3-4.Amongst post-graduate participants, 39(86.7) participants had TW ranging from 2-3, 6(13.3%) participants had TW ranging from 3-4. A significantly significant relationship was discovered between status of education of a person and TW when value of significance came out to be 0.000. (Table-14, Graph-15)

DISTRIBUTION OF STUDY PARTICIPANTS AS PER DENTAL VISITS

Amongst study population of 630 participants, 42(6.7%) participants had a dental visit in last 6 months, 82(13%) participants had a dental visit between 6 months to 1 year, 200(31.7%) participants had a dental visit in past 1-2 years, 149(23.7%) participants had a dental visit more than 2 years back, 157(24.9%) participants denied that they had dental visits in past few years. (Table-6, Graph-6)

ASSOCIATION OF STUDY SUBJECTS WITH DENTAL VISITS ON TEETH-WEAR

Amongst the study population, those participants who visited any dental clinic during the last 6 months, 5(11.9%) participants had TW ranging from 1-2, 37(88.1%) participants had TW ranging from 2-3, amongst those who visited any dental clinic during the last 6 months-1 year, 35(42.7%) participants had TW ranging from 1-2, 35(42.7%) participants had TW ranging from 2-3, 12(14.6%) participants had TW ranging from 3-4. Amongst those who visited any dental clinic during the last 1-2 year, 51(25.5%) participants had TW ranging from 1-2, 143(71.5%) participants had TW ranging from 2-3, and 6 (3%) participants had TW ranging from 3-4. Amongst those who haven't visited any dental clinic since last 2 years, 52(34.9%) participants had TW ranging from 1-2, 91(61.1%) participants had TW ranging from 2-3, 6(4%) participants had TW ranging from 3-4, amongst those who have never visited any dental clinic, 66(42%) participants had TW ranging from 1-2, 91(58%) participants had TW ranging from 2-3. A significantly significant relationship was discovered between last visit to a dentist of a person and TW when value of significance came out to be 0.000. (Table-14, Graph-16)

DISTRIBUTION OF STUDY PARTICIPANTS AS PER REASON FOR DENTAL VISIT

Amongst study population of 630 participants, 101(16%) participants visited a dentist for general check-up, 371(58.9%) participants visited a dentist for some specific treatment while 158(25.1%) participants denied for either of them. (Table-7, Graph-7)

ASSOCIATION OF STUDY SUBJECTS WITH REASON FOR DENTAL VISITS ON TEETH-WEAR

Amongst the study population, those participants who visited dental clinic for general check-up, 17(16.8%) participants had TW ranging from 1-2, 84(83.2%) participants had TW ranging from 2-3.Amongst the study population, those participants who visited dental clinic for specific treatment, 131(35.3%) participants had TW ranging from 1-2, 216(58.2%) participants had TW ranging from 2-3, 24(6.5%) participants had TW ranging from 3-4. A significantly significant relationship was discovered between reason of visit to a dentist of a person and TW when value of significance came out to be 0.000. (Table-14, Graph-16)

DISTRIBUTION OF STUDY PARTICIPANTS AS PER ORAL HYGIENE AIDS USED

Amongst study population of 630 participants, 417(66.2%) participants used toothbrush as oral hygiene aid, 196(31.1%) participants used fingers as oral hygiene aid, and 17 (2.7%) participants used tree stick as oral hygiene aid. (Table-8, Graph-8)

ASSOCIATION OF STUDY SUBJECTS AS PER ORAL HYGIENE AIDS ON TEETH-WEAR

Amongst the study population, those participants who used toothbrush as oral hygiene aid,143(34.3%) participants had TW ranging from 1-2, 25.6(61.4%) participants had TW ranging from 2-3, 18(4.3%) participants had TW ranging from 3-4.Amongst the study population, those participants who used finger as oral hygiene aid, 61(31.1%) participants had TW ranging from 1-2, 129(65.8%) participants had TW ranging from 2-3, 6(3.1%) participants had TW ranging from 3-4.Amongst the study population, those participants who used tree stick as oral hygiene aid, 5(29.4%) participants had TW ranging from 1-2, 12(70.6%) participants had TW ranging from 2-3. A non significant relationship was discovered between aids of oral hygiene used by a person and TW when value of significance came out to be 0.686. (Table 14, Graph-16)

DISTRIBUTION OF STUDY PARTICIPANTS AS PER ORAL HYGIENE MATERIAL USED

Amongst study population of 630 participants, 363(57.6%) participants used toothpaste as oral hygiene material, 250(39.7%) participants used toothpowder, and 11 (1.7%) participants used charcoal while just 6 (1%) participants used salt as oral hygiene material. (Table-9, Graph-9)

ASSOCIATION OF STUDY SUBJECTS AS PER ORAL HYGIENE MATERIAL ON TEETH-WEAR

Amongst the study population, those participants who used toothpaste as oral hygiene material,104(28.7%) participants had TW ranging from 1-2, 235(64.7%) participants had TW ranging from 2-3, and 24 (6.6%) participants had TW ranging from 3-4.Amongst the study population, those participants who used tooth powder as oral hygiene material , 100(40%) participants had TW ranging from 1-2, 150(60%) participants had TW ranging from 2-3.Amongst the study population, those participants who used charcoal as oral hygiene material, 5(45.5%) participants had TW ranging from 1-2, 6(54.5%) participants had TW ranging from 2-3.Amongst the study population, those participants who used salt as oral hygiene material, only 6(100%) participants had TW ranging from 2-3. A significantly significant relationship was discovered between material of oral hygiene used by a person and TW when value of significance came out to be 0.001. (Table-14, Graph-16)

DISTRIBUTION OF STUDY PARTICIPANTS AS PER FREQUENCY OF BRUSHING

Amongst study population of 630 participants, 387(61.4%) participants brushed their teeth only once, 178(28.3%) brushed their teeth twice daily while 65(10.3%) participants brushed their teeth thrice daily. (Table-10, Graph-10)

ASSOCIATION OF STUDY SUBJECTS AS PER FREQUENCY OF BRUSHING ON TEETH-WEAR

Amongst the study population, those participants who brushed their teeth once daily, 145(37.5%) participants had TW ranging from 1-2, 230(59.4%) participants had TW ranging from 2-3, and 12(3.1%) participants had TW ranging from 3-4.Amongst the study population, those participants who brushed their teeth twice daily, 54(30.3%) participants had TW ranging from 1-2, 112(62.9%) participants had TW ranging from 2-3, and 12(6.7%) participants had TW ranging from 3-4.Amongst the study population, those participants who brushed their teeth thrice daily, 10(15.4%) participants had TW ranging from 1-2, 55(84.6%) participants had TW ranging from 2-3. A significantly significant relationship was discovered between brushing frequency of a person and TW when value of significance came out to be 0.000. (Table-14, Graph-17)

DISTRIBUTION OF STUDY PARTICIPANTS AS PER CONSUMPTION OF FRUIT/CITRIC DRINKS

Amongst study population of 630 participants, 360(57.1%) participants agreed that they consumed fruit/citric drinks, 270(42.9%) participants denied that they consumed fruit/citric drinks. (Table-11, Graph-11)

ASSOCIATION OF STUDY SUBJECTS AS PER CONSUMPTION OF FRUIT/CITRIC DRINKS ON TEETH-WEAR

Amongst the study population those who consumed fruit/citric drinks,96(26.7%) participants had TW ranging from 1-2, 246(68.3%) participants had TW ranging from 2-3, and 18(5%) participants had TW ranging from 3-4. Amongst the study population those who didn't consumed fruit/citric drinks, 113(41.9%) participants had TW ranging from 1-2, 151(55.9%) participants had TW ranging from 2-3, and 6(2.2%) participants had TW ranging from 3-4. A significantly significant relationship was discovered between intakes of citric or fruit drinks of a person and TW when value of significance came out to be 0.000. (Table-14, Graph-17)

DISTRIBUTION OF STUDY PARTICIPANTS AS PER CONSUMPTION OF BEVERAGES/CARBONATED DRINKS

Amongst study population of 630 participants, 360(47.9%) participants agreed that they consumed beverages/carbonated drinks, 270(52.1%) participants denied that they consumed beverages/carbonated drinks. (Table-12, Graph-12)

ASSOCIATION OF STUDY SUBJECTS AS PER CONSUMPTION OF BEVERAGES/CARBONATED DRINKS ON TEETH-WEAR

Amongst the study population those who consumed beverages/carbonated drinks, 91(30.1%) participants had TW ranging from 1-2, 187(61.9%) participants had TW ranging from 2-3, and

24(7.9%) participants had TW ranging from 3-4. Amongst the study population those who didn't consumed beverages/carbonated drinks, 118(36%) participants had TW ranging from 1-2, 210(64%) participants had TW ranging from 2-3. A significantly significant relationship was discovered between intakes of drinks which are carbonated or the beverages intake of a person and TW when value of significance came out to be 0.000. (Table-14, Graph-17)

DISTRIBUTION OF STUDY PARTICIPANTS AS PER BRUSHING TECHNIQUE

Amongst study population of 630 participants, 392(62.2%) participants told that they brushed their teeth horizontally, 164(26%) participants told that they brushed their teeth vertically, 74(11.7%) participants told that they used a combination of both horizontal and vertical movements for brushing their teeth. (Table-13, Graph-13)

ASSOCIATION OF STUDY SUBJECTS AS PER BRUSHING TECHNIQUE ON TEETH-WEAR

Amongst study population, those who brushed their teeth horizontally, 136(34.7%) participants had TW ranging from 1-2, 238(60.7%) participants had TW ranging from 2-3, and 18(4.6%) participants had TW ranging from 3-4. Amongst study population, those who brushed their teeth vertically, 52(31.7%) participants had TW ranging from 1-2, 106(64.6%) participants had TW ranging from 2-3, and 6(3.7%) participants had TW ranging from 3-4. Amongst study population, those who brushed their teeth both horizontally and vertically, 21(28.4%) participants had TW ranging from 1-2, 53(71.6%) participants had TW ranging from 2-3. A non significant relationship was discovered between technique of doing brushing employed by a person and TW when value of significance came out to be 0.231. (Table-14 Graph-17)

CORRELATION BETWEEN TEETH WEAR AND OHRQoL

Amongst those participants those who had TW ranging between1 to 2, amongst them majority (77%) had mild impact on OHRQoL followed by 45(21.5%) having no impact on OHRQoL, followed by 2(1%) having moderate impact on OHRQoL, followed by 1(0.5%) participant having severe impact on OHRQoL. Amongst those participants those who had TW ranging between 2 to 3, amongst them majority (92.4%) had mild impact on OHRQoL followed by 23(5.8%) having no impact on OHRQoL, followed by 6(1.5%) having moderate impact on OHRQoL, followed by 1(0.3%) participant having severe impact on OHRQoL. Amongst those participants those who had TW ranging between 3 to 4, amongst them majority (87.5%) had mild impact on OHRQoL, followed by 2(8.3%) having moderate impact on OHRQoL, followed by 1(4.2%) participant having severe impact on OHRQoL. If we talk about teeth wear overall, 549(87.1%) participants had mild impact on OHRQoL, followed by 68(10.8%) participants having no impact on OHRQoL, followed by 10(1.6%) participants having moderate impact on OHRQoL, followed by 3(0.5%) participants having severe impact on OHRQoL. Thus we can say that a significantly significant relationship was discovered between TW and OHRQoL when value of significance came out to be 0.001. (Table-15, Graph-18)

Also amongst all the domains of OHIP-14, physical pain was the most affected domain followed by physical disability. A highly and significantly significant relationship was discovered between TW and all domains of OHIP-14 translated version when value of significance came out to be 0.001. (Table -16).

TABLES

1. PARTICIPANTS DISTRIBUTION ON BASIS OF GENDER IN POPULATION

Subjects	Frequency	Percent

| Male | 343 | 54.4 |
| Female | 287 | 45.6 |

2. AGE DISTRIBUTION OF STUDY PARTICIPANTS

Subjects	Frequency	Percent
35	52	8.3%
36	60	9.5%
37	69	11%
38	103	16.3%
39	62	9.8%
40	86	13.7%
41	49	7.8%
42	70	11.1%
43	39	6.2%
44	34	5.4%
45	6	1%

3. DISTRIBUTION OF STUDY PARTICIPANTS AS PER SOCIOECONOMIC STATUS

Subjects	Frequency	Percentage
Upper class	42	6.7%
Upper middle class	88	14%
Lower middle class	222	35.2%

Upper Lower class	205	32.5%
Lower class	73	11.6%

4. DISTRIBUTION OF STUDY PARTICIPANTS AS PER PLACE OF RESIDENCE

Subjects	Frequency	Percentage
Village	159	25.2%
City	471	74.8%

5. DISTRIBUTION OF STUDY PARTICIPANTS AS PER EDUCATIONAL QUALIFICATIONS

Subjects	Frequency	Percentage
10th pass	57	9%
12th pass	144	22.9%
Graduation	384	61%
Post-graduation	45	7.1%

6. DISTRIBUTION OF STUDY PARTICIPANTS AS PER DENTAL VISITS

Subjects	Frequency	Percentage
Last 6 months	42	6.7%
Last 6 months-1 year	82	13%
1-2 year	200	31.7%
More than 2 year	149	23.7%

None	157	24.9%

7. DISTRIBUTION OF STUDY PARTICIPANTS AS PER REASON FOR DENTAL VISITS

Subjects	Frequency	Percentage
General check-up	101	16%
Specific treatment	371	58.9%
None	158	25.1%

8. DISTRIBUTION OF STUDY PARTICIPANTS AS PER ORAL HYGIENE AIDS USED

Subjects	Frequency	Percentage
Toothbrush	417	66.2%
Finger	196	31.1%
Tree-stick	17	2.7%

9. DISTRIBUTION OF STUDY PARTICIPANTS AS PER ORAL HYGIENE MATERIAL USED

Subjects	Frequency	Percentage
Toothpaste	363	57.6%
Toothpowder	250	39.7%
Charcoal	11	1.7%
Salt	6	1%

10. DISTRIBUTION OF STUDY PARTICIPANTS AS PER FREQUENCY OF BRUSHING

Subjects	Frequency	Percentage
Once	387	61.4%
Twice	178	28.3%
Thrice	65	10.3%

11. DISTRIBUTION OF STUDY PARTICIPANTS AS PER CONSUMPTION OF FRUIT/CITRIC DRINKS

Subjects	Frequency	Percentage
Yes	360	57.1%
No	270	42.9%

12. DISTRIBUTION OF STUDY PARTICIPANTS AS PER CONSUMPTION OF BEVERAGES/CARBONATED DRINKS

Subjects	Frequency	Percentage
Yes	302	47.9%
No	328	52.1%

13. DISTRIBUTION OF STUDY PARTICIPANTS AS PER BRUSHING TECHNIQUE

Subjects	Frequency	Percentage
Horizontal	392	62.2%

Vertical	164	26%
Combination	74	11.7%

14. ASSOCIATION BETWEEN TEETH WEAR AND OTHER FACTORS

PARAMETERS		TEETH WEAR (1-2)	TEETH WEAR (2-3)	TEETH WEAR (3-4)	Chi-square value	P value
Gender	Male	97	228	18	10.954	0.004
		28.27%	66.47%	5.24%		(sig)
	Female	112	169	6		
		39.02%	58.88%	2.09%		
Age	35	23	29	0	90.927	0.001
		44.2%	55.8%	0%		(sig)
	36	28	32	0		
		46.7%	53.3%	0%		
	37	23	40	6		
		33.3%	58%	8.7%		
	38	35	56	12		
		34%	54.4%	11.7%		
	39	32	30	0		
		51.6%	48.4%	0%		

	40	15	71	0		
		17.4%	82.6%	0%		
	41	12	37	0		
		24.5%	75.5%	0%		
	42	30	34	6		
		42.9%	48.6%	8.6%		
	43	5	34	0		
		12.8%	87.2%	0%		
	44	6	28	0		
		17.6%	82.4%	0%		
	45	0	6	0		
		0%	100%	0%		
Social and economical condition	Range of Upper class	5	37	0	62.90	0.002
		11.9%	88.1%	0%	4	(sig)
	Range of Upper middle class	41	35	12		
		46.6%	39.8%	13.6%		
	Range of Lower middle class	56	160	6		
		25.2%	72.1%	2.7%		
	Range of Upper lower class	84	115	6		
		41%	56.1%	2.9%		
	Range of Lower class	23	50	0		
		31.5%	68.5%	0%		
Place of	Village	55	92	12	8.824	0.012

residence		34.6%	57.9%	7.5%		(NS)
	City	154	305	12		
		32.7%	64.8%	2.5%		
Educational qualification	10th pass	17	40	0	45.17	0.000
		29.8%	70.2%	0%	1	(sig)
	12th pass	67	71	6		
		46.5%	49.3%	4.2%		
	Graduation	125	247	12		
		32.6%	64.3%	3.1%		
	Post graduation	0	39	6		
		0%	86.7%	13.3%		
Last dental visit	Last 6 months	5	37	0	61.11	0.000
		11.9%	88.1%	0%	2	(sig)
	6 months – 1 year	35	35	12		
		42.7%	42.7%	14.6%		
	1-2 year	51	143	6		
		25.5%	71.5%	3%		
	More than 2 year	52	91	6		
		34.9%	61.1%	4%		
	None	66	91	0		
		42%	58%	0%		

Reason for visit to dental clinic	General check-up	17	84	0	34.37	0.000
		16.8%	83.2%	0%	1	(sig)
	Specific treatment	131	216	24		
		35.3%	58.2%	6.5%		
	None	61	97	0		
		38.6%	61.4%	0%		
Oral hygiene aid used	Toothbrush	143	25.6	18	2.269	0.686
		34.3%	61.4%	4.3%		(NS)
	Finger	61	129	6		
		31.1%	65.8%	3.1%		
	Tree-stick	5	12	0		
		29.4%	70.6%	0%		
Oral hygiene material used	Toothpaste	104	235	24	27.85	0.001
		28.7%	64.7%	6.6%	3	(sig)
	Tooth powder	100	150	0		
		40%	60%	0%		
	Charcoal	5	6	0		
		45.5%	54.5%	0%		
	Salt	0	6	0		
		0	100%	0%		
Frequency of brushing	Once	145	230	12	21.38	0.000
		37.5%	59.4%	3.1%	2	(sig)
	Twice	54	112	12		

		30.3%	62.9%	6.7%		
	Thrice	10	55	0		
		15.4%	84.6%	0%		
Consumption of fruit/citric acids	Yes	96	246	18	17.618	0.000 (sig)
		26.7%	68.3%	5%		
	No	113	151	6		
		41.9%	55.9%	2.2%		
Consumption of beverages/carbonated drinks	Yes	91	187	24	27.795	0.000 (sig)
		30.1%	61.9%	7.9%		
	No	118	210	0		
		36%	64%	0%		
Brushing technique	Horizontal	136	238	18	5.618	0.231 (NS)
		34.7%	60.7%	4.6%		
	Vertical	52	106	6		
		31.7%	64.6%	3.7%		
	Combination	21	53	0		
		28.4%	71.6%	0%		

15. ASSOCIATION BETWEEN TEETH WEAR AND OHRQoL

Teeth wear	OHIP			Chi square value	p-value

	No impact range (from zero till 14)	Mild range (from 15 till 28)	Moderate range (from 29 till 32)	Severe range (from 33 till 56)	52.545	0.001 (sig)
TW 1-2	45(21.5%)	161(77%)	2(1%)	1(0.5%)		
TW 2-3	23(5.8%)	367(92.4%)	6(1.5%)	1(0.3%)		
TW 3-4	0(0%)	21(87.5%)	2(8.3%)	1(4.2%)		
Total	68(10.8%)	549(87.1%)	10(1.6%)	3(0.5%)		

16. MEAN OHIP-14 DOMAIN SCORES AND ITS IMPACT IN RELATION TO SEVERITY OF TEETH WEAR AMONG THE STUDIED POPULATION

Teeth wear severity	Functional limitation	Physical pain	Psychological discomfort	Physical disability	Psychological disability	Social disability	Handicap	Overall OHIP
1-2	2.51±0.659	2.56±0.913	2.45±0.671	2.48±0.872	2.3±0.67	2.41±0.66	2.46±0.63	17.17±4.005
2-3	2.76±0.	3.06±0.	2.94±0.71	3.02±0.	2.7±0.75	2.75±0.	2.84±0.	20.09±

	68	944	6	738		74	74	3.84
3-4	3.38±0.97	3.71±0.908	3.5±1.06	3.38±1.173	3.13±1.3	3.33±1.09	3±1.3	23.42±7.16
Overall score	2.7±0.7	2.92±0.972	2.8±0.76	2.86±0.84	2.59±0.79	2.66±0.76	2.72±0.76	19.25±4.36
p value	0.000 (sig.)	0.000 (sig.)	0.000 (sig.)	0.000 (sig.)	0.000 (sig.)	0.000 (sig.)	0.000 (sig.)	0.000 (sig.)

GRAPHS -

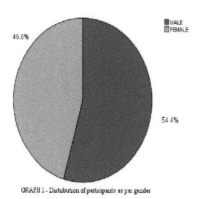

GRAPH 1 - Distribution of participants as per gender

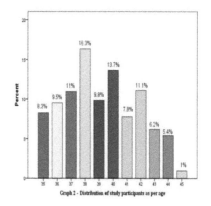

Graph 2 - Distribution of study participants as per age

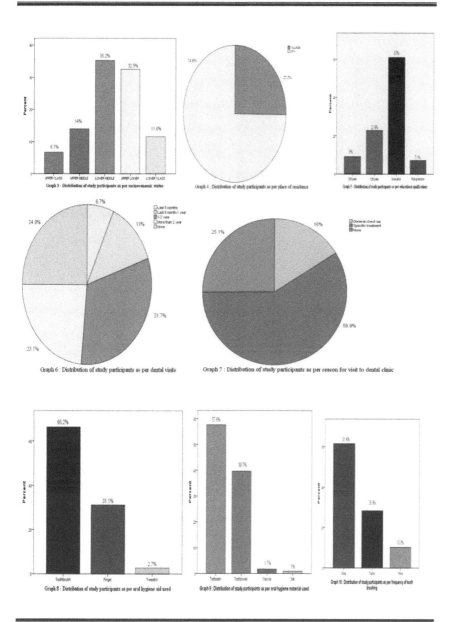

Graph 3 - Distribution of study participants as per socioeconomic status

Graph 4 : Distribution of study participants as per place of residence

Graph 5 : Distribution of study participants as per educational qualification

Graph 6 : Distribution of study participants as per dental visits

Graph 7 : Distribution of study participants as per reason for visit to dental clinic

Graph 8 : Distribution of study participants as per oral hygiene aid used

Graph 9 : Distribution of study participants as per oral hygiene material used

Graph 10 : Distribution of study participants as per frequency of tooth brushing

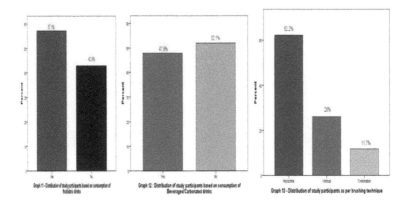

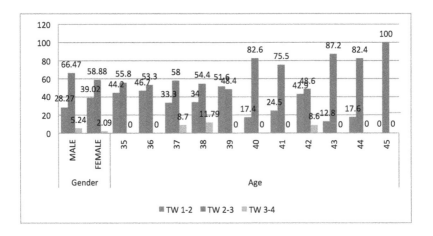

Graph 14 – Association between teeth wear and other factors

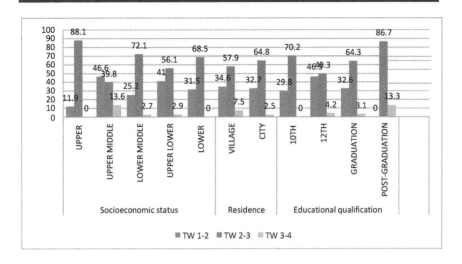

Graph 15 – Association between teeth wear and other factors

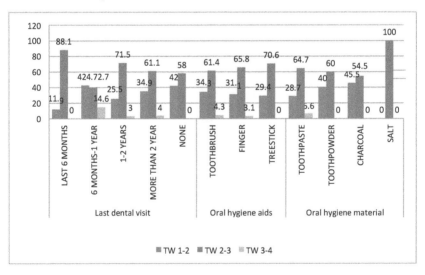

Graph 16 – Association between teeth wear and other factors

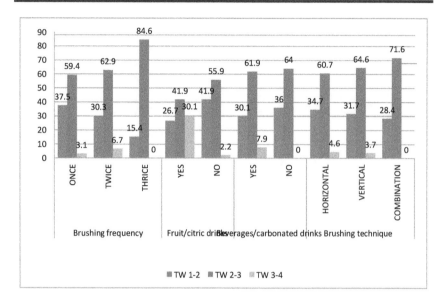

Graph 17 – Association between teeth wear and other factors

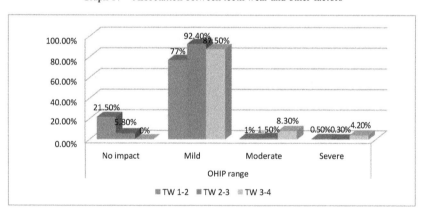

Graph 18– Association between teeth wear and OHIP range

DISCUSSION

Teeth wear is becoming a very common problem amongst both the younger and older adults worldwide. Etiology of it is multifactorial hence we can't designate one single factor for its etiology. As per some studies TW is caused to habits of a person and as per some studies TW's etiology is designated to the type of diet a person takes. In our study we correlated TW with OHRQoL and there came up a positive correlation between TW and OHRQoL. As per a study conducted by Al Omiri et al[9] the age and gender showed no association with TW while as per our study TW was positively associated with age and gender of a population.

As per a study conducted by Smith et al[10] in which they assessed TW and its etiological factors, tooth brushing frequency showed a positive correlation with TW. Those who brushed twice daily had most TW which was same as our inference as in our study too TW was very significantly associated with brushing frequency. As per a study conducted by Ahmed H et al[11] to assess relation between NCCLs and its etiological factors, there came out to be a negative correlation between NCCLs and age while in our study there was a significant relation between age and TW.

As per a study conducted by Wang P et al[12] on children's TW and its associated etiologies, mother's level of education showed a positive correlation with the erosion i.e. those who had highly educated mothers, those children had less erosion chances, and in our study the level of education of a person showed a very high correlation with the TW. In their study erosion was positively associated with the amount of carbonated drinks a person takes which was same as the inference of our study.

As per a study conducted by Barlett et al[13] on TW and associated risk factors, there came out to be non significant association between TW and the frequency of intake of carbonated drinks while in our study there was a significant and a positive relation between intake of beverages and carbonated drinks and TW. As per a study conducted by Al Zarea et al[14] on TW, most common risk factors associated with TW came out to be acidic food and drinks which was also in line with the inference of our cross sectional study.

As per a study conducted by Papagianni CE et al[15] on TW, results concluded that TW was directly linked with OHRQoL which was as the same inference in our study too. As per a study conducted by Barlett et al[16] on TW, they concluded that BEW was directly associated with age and this was the same as the inference of our cross sectional study too. According to their study gender showed no association with BEW, while in our study gender showed a positive correlation with TW. As per a study conducted by Kumar S et al[17] on children assessing their TW, it was concluded that thelocation of living of that child be it rural or urban isn't associated with TW, which was same as the inference of our study conducted on the adults of age group 35-44 years.

As per a study conducted by Abanto et al[19] on children aged 6-14 years assessing their erosion, age, gender, dental caries, frequency of juice intake and the family income were just not associated with TW. While in our study which was conducted on adults aged 35-44 years all these factors were positively associated with the level of TW in a person. As per a study conducted by Pradeep Y et al[22] assessing their oral health majority of participants were in consent with the fact that oral health of their oral cavity is very well linked to the QoL of theirs which was in consent with our inference related to OHRQoLthat our population's TW which was a factor impacting oral health affected OHRQoL.

As per a study conducted by Kumar S et al[23] on TW it was assessed that gender of a person, socioeconomic status of a person, oral hygiene material a person uses and frequency of tooth brushing, frequency of dental visits of a person, intake of carbonated drinks in a person's routine have got no impact on the TW a person has, as per their study the factors that were associated with TW were the oral hygiene material used by a person and the technique of brushing implemented by a person, while in our study though the oral hygiene material used by a person showed a positive correlation with TW but the technique of brushing implemented by a person in his/her daily routine showed no relation with TW. As per a study conducted by Hegde MN et al[24] on TW, males seemed to have more TW as compared to females in that population which was same as in our population's results because in our study too, males seemed to have more TW as compared to females. As per a study conducted by Deshpande S[25] who conducted a study to assess the TW in a population, came up with a conclusion that most TW that occurred in that population was of the grade 2 , which was same as the inference of our study's assessment.

As per a study conducted by Andrade et al[26] on TW it was assessed that TW came out to have a positive association with age which was in line with the inference of our study in which also there was a positive correlation between age of a person and TW. As per a study conducted by Li MHM[28] et al on TW correlating with OHRQoL, it was assessed that as TW was increasing in that population so was their value of OHIP increasing in that population, which was the same result as we concluded from our study that as TW was increasing so was the level and value of OHIP was increasing.

As per a study conducted by Antunes et al[29] on TW in children, there was no significant association between socioeconomic status of those children and the level of TW they had in their oral cavity while in our study which was conducted in adults there was a positive correlation between TW and socioeconomic status of that population. As per a study conducted by Vidyadhar MSB et al[31] on adults regarding their TW it was concluded that their diet was the main reason for their etiology of TW while in our study not only dietary habits and dietary patterns but many other reasons also led to TW in that population including their socioeconomic status, their pattern of oral hygiene, their habits related to oral hygiene, also played a major role.

As per a study conducted by Allaq et al[32] regarding TW in a population it was assessed that TW is directly linked to the age of that population which was in line with our study's inference. As per a study conducted by Praveena J et al[33] regarding TW in a population and its association with OHRQoL with the help of OHIP it was assessed that OHIP's all domains were significantly associated with TW except the domain of functional limitation while in our study in which we correlated TW with OHRQoL with the help of Hindi translated version of OHIP-14, we assessed that all domains of OHIP-14 were significantly associated with OHRQoL including functional limitation.

As per a study conducted by Hegde MN et al[34] on adults regarding their TW, it was assessed that males had more TW as compared to females in that population which was in line with our study's assessment too. They also concluded that those who belonged to urban location had more TW while in our study the place of residence had no significant relation with TW.

As per a study conducted by Kumar A et al[36] in which erosion of a population was assessed and further it was concluded that erosion showed a positive correlation with the OHRQoL i.e. as the erosion was increasing so the OHRQoL was decreasing and the OHIP value was increasing in that population. As per a study conducted by Mehta SB et al[37] amongst adults who were assessed for their erosion by BEWE and its association with OHIP, it was concluded that as BEWE score was increasing so was their OHIP score hence it showed a positive correlation with it. As per a study conducted by Patel J et al[38] amongst adults TW showed indirect association with

OHRQoL. Though those who had moderate and severe TW, they showed a positive association with the OHRQoL, which was not as per our study's conclusion. As per a study conducted by Khalifa et al[39] amongst adults regarding their TW, it was assessed that gender of that population and their socioeconomic status showed a positive correlation with TW. As per a study conducted by Soares et al[40] amongst adults regarding their TW, it was assessed that their TW was directly associated with OHIP value and amongst all the domains of OHIP.

As per a study conducted by Kalsi H et al[41] amongst a population it was assessed that as the age was increasing the BEWE value was also increasing, while in our study we took only the age group of 35-44 aged people and also concluding that there is a positive correlation between age and TW. As per a study conducted by Penoni DC et al[42] amongst a population regarding their NCCLs, it was assessed that males had a higher frequency Of NCCLs. Especially those males who were elder in age and those who had harmful brushing habits showed a higher frequency of NCCLs. This inference was quite related to our study's inference too as in our population also males were having more TW and their oral hygiene habits affected their TW too.

As per a study conducted by Kannan A et al[43] regarding their TW it was assessed that TW was directly associated with the consumption of acidic beverages and those who consumed these beverages on a regular basis had lower OHRQoL. This finding was seen in our study too but in their study it was seen that as TW was increasing its impact on OHIP was limited but in our study TW had a direct association with OHIP. As per a study conducted by Lim SN et al[44] on TW assessment in a population of military workers it was assessed that TW was directly associated with the intake of acidic content of a person and intake of carbonated drinks which was the same inference we drawn from our study.

CONCLUSION

TW is multifactorial and a complex lesion. It has become a matter of public health concern in both the developed and the developing countries. It has become a risk factor in those individuals who have a regular habit of having frequent intake of beverages, carbonated drinks, alcohol, fr4uit drinks, and citric acid based drinks.

The main aim of this study was to find the extent of impact of TW on an individual's day to day living and on oral health and further reduce the impact. With the scope and limitations of this study mentioned, it has thus been concluded that TW has got a direct association and a positive correlation with the OHRQoL. As TW was increasing, so were the OHIP values, which indicated a lesser OHRQoL. The study also gives us the information that how maintaining a regular and a healthy dietary lifestyle and oral hygiene can help us to combat from being affected by TW. This was also noticed that those who belonged from a comparatively lower socioeconomic status and lower educational background tend to have more TW, hence poorer OHRQoL.

Prevalence of TW in the population was high amongst those who had intake of alcohol/beverages/fruit drinks/citric drinks. Thus this is one of the most common etiological factors for causation of TW.

Hence it was the need of the hour for adults to have a regular visit to a dentist so that their lesions could be identified earlier which further stops their OHRQoL to worsen hence helping them to maintain a proper healthy lifestyle. General dental care can also be achieved through regular dental visits which is helpful in avoiding this lesion on a long term basis. TW can't be reversed but its further degradation can be prevented by monitoring the etiological causes.

From our study we conclude that 35-44 years age group participants tend to be more affected by TW. Hence dental care professionals should be concerned on how to assess complete oral examination in these individuals and make them aware about the severity of TW. Early detection of this lesion can help in reducing the severe effects of TW in a population. Although the main or the exact causative or etiological factor can't be described in a single term as this lesion is multifactorial.

As a public health dentist it is ought to be our responsibility to reduce the burden of this lesion by educating the masses, making them adapt to healthy lifestyle practices and to healthy oral hygiene practices too and helping them modify their diet and dietary patterns in a healthy way so that they can lead a happy and productive life and their OHRQoL as well as their QoL won't be affected. Efforts should be taken to monitor, reduce and prevent the habits and uptake of all the etiological factors that are associated with TW and to beforehand make the population aware about the same. Also population should be made aware regarding the risk of neglecting treatment of TW and its further possible consequences on both the oral and general health of that individual. Necessary educational and awareness programs must be mandatorily conducted so that the population is made aware of the consequences and so that there is improvement in the community and public health importance related to the etiology, prevention and results of TW on oral and general health overall.

LIMITATIONS

- The study is cross sectional in design so it doesn't investigate the effect and cause relationship
- The results of this particular cross sectional study can't be generalized as we only took a section of population of adults belonging to age group of 35-44 years.

RECOMMENDATIONS

Teeth wear can now be considered as one of those neglected issues which are affecting the society all over the world. It also has a very prominent effect on the OHRQoL and thus on QoL of an individual and of the society as well.

Following recommendations are given –

- Health awareness programs with proper monitored actions regarding awareness regarding teeth wear etiology must be conducted
- Encouragement and motivation should be given by various dental practitioners and medical practitioners too to increase the quality and to improve the oral health so that the risk of teeth wear can be decreased.
- As intake of alcohol, beverages, fruit drinks, citric drinks had a major role in the etiology of TW, there should be proper awareness programs conducted to make people aware regarding their monitored uptake in their day to day life.
- Further encouragement of healthy lifestyle amongst all the individuals of a society so that the load of this particular lesion will be reduced
- Public health dentist plays an important role in preventing this lesion at both the individual and community basis
- Further analytical studies are recommended with a larger sample size for a more detailed analysis.

BIBLIOGRAPHY

1. Ramalho A, Miranda J. The relationship between wear and dissipated energy in sliding systems. Wear. 2006; 260:361–367.

2. Mair L, Stolarski T, Vowles R, Lloyd C. Wear : mechanisms, manifestations and measurement. Report of a workshop. J Dent. 1996; 24:141–148.

3. LEE, He LH, Lyons K, Swain MV. Tooth wear and wear investigations in dentistry. Journal of oral rehabilitation.2012;39:217-225

4. Bartlett DW. The role of erosion in tooth wear: aetiology, prevention and management. Int Dent J. 2005; 55:277–284.

5. Arnadottir IB, Holbrook WP, Eggertsson H, Gudmundsdottir H, Jonsson SH Gudlaugsson JO et al. Prevalence of dental erosion in children: a national survey. Comm Dent Oral Epidemiol. 2010; 38:521–526.

6. Mahalick J, Knap F, Weiter E. Occlusal wear in prosthodontics. J Am Dent Assoc. 1971;82:154–159.

7. Hudson J, Goldstein G, Georgescu M. Enamel wear caused by three different restorative materials. J Prosthet Dent. 1995; 74:647–654.

8. Frias F J L, Cosano L C, Gonzalez J M, Carreras J M L, Egea J J S, Clinical measurement of tooth wear:tooth wear indices. J ClinExp Dent 2012;4(1):e48-53

9. Al-Omiri MK, Lamey PJ, Clifford T. Impact of tooth wear on daily living. Int J Prosthodont. 2006 Nov-Dec; 19(6):601-5.

10. Smith WA, Marchan S, Rafeek RN. The prevalence and severity of non-carious cervical lesions in a group of patients attending a university hospital in Trinidad. J Oral Rehabil. 2008 Feb; 35(2):128-34.

11. Ahmed H, Sadaf D, Rahman M. Factors associated with Non-carious cervical lesions(NCCLs) in teeth.Journal of the College of Physicians and Surgeons Pakistan 2009, Vol. 19 (5): 279-282

12. Wang P, Lin HC, Chen JH,Liang HY. The prevalence of dental erosion and associated risk factors in 12-13 year old school children in southern china. BMC Public health.2010;10

13. Barlett DW, Fares J, Shirodaria S, Chiu K, Ahmad N, Sherriff M. The association of tooth wear, diet and dietary habits in adults aged 18-30 years old. Journal of dentistry.2011; 39:811-816.

14. Al-Zarea BK. Tooth surface loss and associated risk factors in northern saudi arabia. ISRN Dent. 2012; 2012:161565

15. Papagianni CE, van der Meulen MJ, Naeije M, Lobbezoo F. Oral health-related quality of life in patients with tooth wear. Journal of oral rehabilitation. 2013; 40(3):185-190.

16. Barlett DW,Lussi A,West NX,Bouchard P,Sanz M,Bourgeois D. Prevalence of tooth wear on buccal and lingual surfaces and possible risk factors in young european adults. J Dent. 2013; 41:1007-1013.

17. Kumar S, Acharya S, Mishra P, Debnath N, Vasthare R. Prevalence and risk factors for dental erosion among 11- to 14-year-old school children in South India. J Oral Sci. 2013; 55(4):329-36.

18. Fotedar S, Sharma KR, Fotedar V, Bharadwaj V, Chauhan A, Manchanda K. Relationship between oral health status and oral health related quality of life in adults attending H.P Government dental college, Shimla, Himachal Pradesh-India. OHDM. 2014; 13(3).

19. Abanto J, Shitsuka C, Murakami C, Ciamponi AL, Raggio DP, Bönecker M. Associated factors to erosive tooth wear and its impact on quality of life in children with cerebral palsy. Special Care in Dentistry. 2014; 34(6):278-285.

20. Liu B, Zhang M, Chen Y, Yao Y. Tooth wear in aging people: an investigation of the prevalence and the influential factors of incisal/occlusal tooth wear in northwest China. BMC Oral Health. 2014 Jun 5;14:65

21. Visscher CM, Lobbezoo F, Schuller AA. Dental status and oral health-related quality of life. A population-based study. Journal of oral rehabilitation. 2014; 41(6):416-422.

22. Pradeep Y, Pushpanjali K. Oral health impact on quality of life assessment among dental patients in Bangalore city. J Indian Assoc Public Health Dent 2014; 12:204-8.

23. Kumar S, Kumar A, Debnath N, Kumar A, K Badiyani B, Basak D, S A Ali M, B Ismail M. Prevalence and risk factors for non-carious cervical lesions in children attending special needs schools in India. J Oral Sci. 2015 Mar; 57(1):37-43 .

24. Hegde MN, Nireeksha.Prevalence of tooth wear due to dietary factors in south canara population.British journal of medicine & medical research. 2015; 9(3):1-6.

25. Deshpande S. Investigation of Tooth Wear and its Associated Etiologies in Adult Patients Visiting Dental Institute in India. Dentistry. 2015;5(1):1-5

26. Andrade FJ, Sales-Peres Ade C, Moura-Grec PG, Mapengo MA, Sales-Peres A, Sales-Peres SH. Nutritional status, tooth wear and quality of life in Brazilian schoolchildren. Public Health Nutr. 2016; 19(8):1479-85.

27. Sanadhya S, Aapaliya P, Jain S, Sharma N, Choudhary G, Dobaria N. Assessment and comparison of clinical dental status and its impact on oral health-related quality of life

among rural and urban adults of Udaipur, India: A cross-sectional study. J Basic Clin Pharma 2015; 6:50-8.

28. Li MHM, Bernabé E. Tooth wear and quality of life among adults in the United Kingdom. J Dent. 2016 Dec;55:48-53

29. Antunes LAA, Castilho T, Marinho M, Fraga RS, Antunes LS. Childhood bruxism: Related factors and impact on oral health-related quality of life. Special Care in Dentistry. 2016; 36(1):7-12.

30. Masood M, Newton T, Bakri NN, Khalid T, Masood Y. The relationship between oral health and oral health related quality of life among elderly people in United Kingdom. Journal of dentistry. 2017; 56:78-83.

31. Vidyadhar MSB, Jain J,Ananda SR. The association of tooth wear, diet and dietary habits among 18-30 year old subjects attending a dental institute in Virajpet, Karnataka. International journal of dental and health sciences.2017;4(3):574-586.

32. Al-Allaq T, Feng C, Saunders RH. Anterior tooth wear and quality of life in a nursing home population. Spec Care Dentist. 2018 ;38(4):187-190

33. Praveena J,Battur H,Fareed N,Khanagar S.The prevalence and impact of teeth wear on oral health related quality of life among rural adult population of Sullia Taluk,D.K. Journal of indian association of public health dentistry.2018 ;16(3).

34. Hegde M, Yelapure M, Honap M, Devadiga D. The prevalence of tooth wear and its associated risk factors in Indian South West coastal population: An epidemiological study. Journal of the International Clinical Dental Research Organization. 2018; 10(1):23-26.

35. Sterenborg BAMM, Bronkhort EM, Wetselaar P, Lobbezoo F, Loomans BAC,Huysmans MC. The influence of management of tooth wear on oral health related quality of life. Clinical Oral Investigations (2018) 22:2567–2573

36. Kumar A , Puranik MP , Sowmya KR , Rajput S.Impact of occupational dental erosion on oral health-related quality of life among battery factory workers in Bengaluru, India. Dental Research Journal. 2019; 16(1):12-17.

37. Mehta SB, Loomans BAC, Banerji S, Bronkhorst EM, Bartlett D. An investigation into the impact of tooth wear on the oral health related quality of life amongst adult dental patients in the United Kingdom, Malta and Australia. J Dent. 2020 Aug;99:103409

38. Patel J, Baker SR. Is toothwear associated with oral health related quality of life in adults in the UK? Community Dental Health. 2020; 37(3):174-179.

39. Al-Khalifa KS. The Prevalence of Tooth Wear in an Adult Population from the Eastern Province of Saudi Arabia. Clin Cosmet Investig Dent. 2020;12:525-531

40. Soares ARDS, Chalub LLFH, Barbosa RS, Campos DE de P, Moreira AN, Ferreira RC. Prevalence and severity of non-carious cervical lesions and dentin hypersensitivity: association with oral-health related quality of life among Brazilian adults. Heliyon. 2021; 7(3):e06492.

41. Kalsi H, Khan A, Bomfim D, Tsakos G, McDonald AV, Rodriguez JM. Quality of life and other psychological factors in patients with tooth wear. British dental journal.2021.

42. Penoni DC, Miranda ME, Sader F, Vettore MV, Leao A. Factors associated with non carious cervical lesions in different age ranges : A cross sectional study. Eur J Dent 2021;15:325–331

43. Kanaan M, Brabant A, Eckert GJ, Hara AT, Carvalho JC. Tooth wear and oral-health-related quality of life in dentate adults. Journal of dentistry. 2022; 125:104269.

44. Lim SN, Tay KJ, Li H, Tan KBC, Tan K. Prevalence and risk factors of erosive tooth wear among young adults in the Singapore military. Clin Oral Investig. 2022 Oct; 26(10):6129-6137.

45. Debnath D J,KakkarR,Modified BG Prasad Socio-economic Classification,Updated-2020.Indian journal of community health 2020;32(01):124-125

46. Smith B G N,Knight J K,An index for measuring the wear of teeth.Br. Dent J 1984;156:435

47. Batra M, Aggarwal V P, Shah A F, Gupta M, Validation of hindi version of oral health impact profile-14 for adults. Journal of Indian association of public health dentistry 2015;13(4);469-474

48. Deshpande NC, Nawathe AA. Translation and validation of Hindi version of Oral Health Impact Profile-14. J Indian Soc Periodontol. 2015 Mar-Apr; 19(2):208-10.

49. Soben Peter. 3rd ed. New Delhi: Arya Publishing house; 2004.Indices in dental epidemiology. Essentials of preventive and community dentistry.

ANNEXURES

ANNEXURE -III

SOCIODEMOGRAPHIC DETAILS

DATE-   OPD NO.-

1.NAME –   2. GENDER-   3. AGE -

4. SES PRASAD'S CLASSIFICATION

a) Upper class b) Upper middle c) Lower middle   d)   Upper lower   e) Lower class

5. PLACE OF RESIDENCE -a) Village   b) City

6. EDUCATIONAL QUALIFICATION

a) 10th pass b) 12th pass   c) Graduation   d) post-graduation

7. WHEN WAS YOUR LAST DENTAL VISIT

a) Last 6 months   b) Last 6 month-1 year   c) 1-2-year d) more than 2 year   e) None

8. REASONS FOR THE VISIT TO DENTAL CLINIC

a) General Check-up   b) Specific Treatment   c) None

9. TYPE OF ORAL HYGIENE AID USED

a) Toothbrush   b) Finger   c) Tree stick

10. ORAL HYGIENE MATERIAL USED

a) Toothpaste   b) Toothpowder   c) Charcoal   d) Salt

11. HOW MANY TIMES DO YOU BRUSH? - a)   Once   b) Twice   c) Thrice

12. CONSUMPTION OF FRUIT/CITRIC DRINKS - a) Yes   b) No

13. CONSUMPTION OF BEVERAGES/CARBONATED DRINKS -a) Yes   b) No

14. BRUSHING TECHNIQUE -a) Horizontal   b) vertical   c) combination

ANNEXURE -IV

SMITH AND KNIGHT TEETH WEAR INDEX

PATIENT NAME-   AGE-   SEX-

UPPER TEETH

8	7	6	5	4	3	2	1	1	2	3	4	5	6	7	8	
																C
																B
																O/I
																L

LOWER TEETH

																L
																O/I
																B
																C
8	7	6	5	4	3	2	1	1	2	3	4	5	6	7	8	

B = buccal or labial

L = lingual or palatal

O = occlusal

I = incisal

C = cervical

0-4 = Tooth wear index score

M = missing

R = restored

ANNEXURE -V

OHIP-14(HINDI) QUESTIONNAIRE

प्रश्नावली:

1. क्या आपको अपने दाँत मुँह, या बत्तिसि की समस्याओं की वजह से लगा कि आपका स्वाद का अहेसास खराब हो गया है?

0= कभी नही	1= शायदही कभी	2= कभी कभी	3= अक्सर	4= बहुत बार

2. क्या आपको मुंह में ददैनाक दर्द हुआ है?

0= कभी नही	1= शायदही कभी	2= कभी कभी	3= अक्सर	4= बहुत बार

3. क्या आपको अपने दाँत, मुँह, या बत्तिसि की समस्याओं की वजह से शब्द उच्चारण मै परेशानी होती है?

0= कभी नही	1= शायदही कभी	2= कभी कभी	3= अक्सर	4= बहुत बार

4. क्या आप अपने दाँत, मुँह ,या बत्तिसिके साथ समस्याओं की वजह से आपका आहार असंतोषजनक रहा है?

0= कभी नहीं	1= शायदही कभी	2= कभी कभी	3= अक्सर	4= बहुत बार

5. क्या आपने दाँत, मुँह, या बत्तिसि के साथ कि समस्याओं की वजह से तनाव महसूस किया है?

0= कभी नहीं	1= शायदही कभी	2= कभी कभी	3= अक्सर	4= बहुत बार

6.क्या आपको अपने दांत, मुंहया बत्तिसि की समस्याओं की वजहसे अपने आपको किसीभी खाद्य पदार्थखाने के लिए असहज पाया है?

0= कभी नहीं	1= शायदही कभी	2= कभी कभी	3= अक्सर	4= बहुत बार

7.क्या आप अपने दाँत, मुँह, या बत्तिसिकी वजह से अपने आपको स्वयंके प्रतिसजग पाया है?

0= कभी नहीं	1= शायदही कभी	2= कभी कभी	3= अक्सर	4= बहुत बार

8.क्या आप अपने दाँत, मुँह, या बत्तिसि के साथ समस्याओं की वजहसे शमिंदा हुए है?

0= कभी नहीं	1= शायदही कभी	2= कभी कभी	3= अक्सर	4= बहुत बार

9.क्या आप अपने दाँत, मुँह, याबत्तिसि के साथ समस्याओं की वजहसे अन्य लोगों के साथ चिड़चिड़ेसे होगये है?

0= कभी नहीं	1= शायदही कभी	2= कभी कभी	3= अक्सर	4= बहुत बार

10.क्या आप अपने दाँत, मुँह, याबत्तिसि के साथ समस्याओं की वजहसे आराम करने में मुश्किल हुई है?

0= कभी नहीं	1= शायदही कभी	2= कभी कभी	3= अक्सर	4= बहुत बार

11. क्या आप अपने दाँत, मुँह, या बत्तिसि के साथ समस्याओं की वजहसे भोजन रोकना पडा है?

0= कभी नहीं	1= शायदही कभी	2= कभी कभी	3= अक्सर	4= बहुत बार

12. क्या आपने महसूस किया है कि सामान्य रूपमें जीवन अपने दाँत, मुँह, याबत्तिसि के साथ समस्याओं की वजह से कम संतोषजनक था?

0= कभी नहीं	1= शायदही कभी	2= कभी कभी	3= अक्सर	4= बहुत बार

13. क्या आप पूरी तरह से अपने दांत, मुंह या बत्तिसिके साथ समस्याओं की वजहसे काम करने में असमर्थहो गये है?

0= कभी नहीं	1= शायदही कभी	2= कभी कभी	3= अक्सर	4= बहुत बार

14. क्या आप अपने दाँत, मुँह, या बत्तिसि के साथ समस्याओं की वजह से अपने सामान्य काम करने में कठिनाई हो रही है?

0= कभी नहीं	1= शायदही कभी	2= कभी कभी	3= अक्सर	4= बहुत बार

OHIP-14 QUESTIONNAIRE (ENGLISH)

NAME-   AGE/SEX-

1) HAVE YOU HAD TROUBLE PRONOUNCING ANY WORDS BECAUSE OF
PROBLEMS WITH YOUR TEETH OR MOUTH

a) Very often   b) fairly often   c) occasionally

d) Hardly ever   e) never

2) HAVE YOU FELT THAT YOUR SENSE OF TASTE HAS WORSENED BECAUSE OF
PROBLEMS WITH TEETH OR MOUTH?

a) Very often   b) fairly often   c) occasionally

d) Hardly ever   e) never

3) HAVE YOU HAD PAINFUL ACHING IN YOUR MOUTH?

a) Very often   b) fairly often   c) occasionally

d) Hardly ever   e) never

4) HAVE YOU FOUND IT UNCOMFORTABLE TO EAT ANY FOODS BECAUSE OF
PROBLEMS WITH YOUR TEETH OR MOUTH?

a) Very often   b) fairly often   c) occasionally

d) Hardly ever   e) never

5) HAVE YOU BEEN SELF CONCIOUS BECAUSE OF TEETH OR MOUTH?

a) Very often   b) fairly often   c) occasionally

d) Hardly ever   e) never

6) HAVE YOU FELT TENSE BECAUSE OF PROBLEMS WITH YOUR TEETH OR
MOUTH?

a)Very often   b) fairly often   c) occasionally

d) Hardly ever   e) never

7) HAS YOUR DIET BEEN UNSATISFACTORY BECAUSE OF PROBLEMS WITH YOUR TEETH OR MOUTH?

a)Very often   b) fairly often   c) occasionally

d) Hardly ever   e) never

8) HAVE YOU HAD TO INTERRUPT MEALS BECAUSE OF PROBLEMS WITH YOUR TEETH OR MOUTH?

a)Very often   b) fairly often   c) occasionally

d) Hardly ever   e) never

9) HAVE YOU FOUND IT DIFFICULT TO RELAX BECAUSE OF PROBLEMS WITH YOUR TEETH OR MOUTH?

a)Very often   b) fairly often   c) occasionally

d) Hardly ever   e) never

10) HAVE YOU BEEN A BIT EMBARRASED BECAUSE OF PROBLEMS WITH YOUR TEETH OR MOUTH?

a)Very often   b) fairly often   c) occasionally

d) Hardly ever   e) never

11) HAVE YOU BEEN A BIT IRRITABLE WITH OTHER PEOPLE BECAUSE OF PROBLEMS WITH YOUR TEETH OR MOUTH?

a)Very often   b) fairly often   c) occasionally

d) Hardly ever   e) never

12) HAVE YOU HAD DIFFICULTY DOING YOUR USUAL JOBS BECAUSE OF PROBLEMS WITH YOUR TEETH OR MOUTH?

a)Very often   b) fairly often   c) occasionally

d) Hardly ever   e) never

13) HAVE YOU FELT THAT LIFE IN GENERAL WAS LESS SATISFYING BECAUSE OF PROBLEMS WITH YOUR TEETH OR MOUTH?

a)Very often   b) fairly often   c) occasionally

d) Hardly ever   e) never

14) HAVE YOU BEEN TOTALLY UNABLE TO FUNCTION BECAUSE OF PROBLEMS WITH YOUR TEETH OR MOUTH?

a)Very often   b) fairly often   c) occasionally

d) Hardly ever   e) never

YOUR KNOWLEDGE HAS VALUE

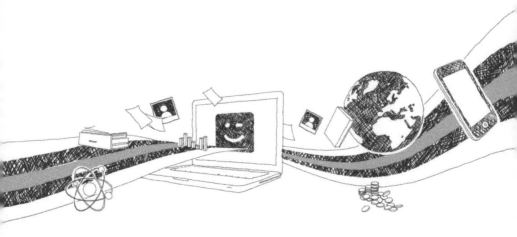

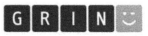